for Jonathan, Caroline and Andrew

the people who
contribute most to my
quality of life

THE QUALITY OF LIFE

The Missing Measurement in Health Care

Lesley Fallowfield

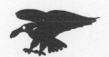

A CONDOR BOOK
SOUVENIR PRESS (E & A) LTD

ISBN 0 285 62942 5 hardback
ISBN 0 285 62952 2 paperback

Photoset, printed and bound in Great Britain by
WBC Bristol and Maesteg

CONTENTS

List of Tables   8
Acknowledgements   10
Preface   13
Introduction   15

1 Philosophical Issues   17
2 Methodological Issues   31
3 The Quality of Life in Cancer   75
4 The Quality of Life in AIDS   114
5 The Quality of Life in Cardiovascular Disease   126
6 The Quality of Life in Arthritis   143
7 The Quality of Life in the Elderly   162
8 The Quality of Dying   186
9 The Health Economist's View of Quality of Life   204

Summary and Conclusion   221
Appendix: Addresses for obtaining tests protected by
    copyright   223
Glossary of medical terms used in text   225
Index   229

LIST OF TABLES

1	Quality of Life	20
2	Things to consider when choosing a test	40
3	The Karnofsky Performance Index	45
4	World Health Organisation Performance Status	47
5	Some definitions and grades for the Katz Index of Activities of Daily Living	48
6	Spitzer's Quality of Life Index	50
7	Some Items from the LASA (Priestman & Baum)	51
8	Part of Selby's LASA	53
9	McGill Pain Questionnaire	54
10	Items from Manitoba Cancer Treatment and Research Foundation Functional Living Index: Cancer (FLIC)	56
11a	Nottingham Health Profile (Part 1)	58
11b	Nottingham Health Profile (Part 2)	59
12	General Health Questionnaire	60
13	Items in the Rotterdam Symptom Checklist (RSCL)	62
14	Some items from Section VI of PAIS	64
15	Some items from Sickness Impact Profile (SIP)	66
16	Part of Profile of Mood States (POMS)	68
17	HAD Scale	69
18	Cancer Survival Statistics	76
19	Psychosocial problems of cancer patients	77
20	The EORTC Lung Cancer Module	97
21	Psychological outcome of mastectomy v. breast conservation	101 102 103
22	Quality of Life after Stroke	135
23	Threats to Quality of Life in Arthritis	147

24   A typical arthritis self-assessment test   148
25   Arthritis Impact Measurement Scale (AIMS)   151
26   Functional Status Index   152
27   Items from Health Assessment Questionnaire
     (HAQ)   153
28   Clifton Assessment Procedures for the Elderly
     (CAPE)   163
29   Assessment areas in the CARE   165
30   People of pensionable age living in Great Britain
     (1981)   174
31a Income of elderly people   175
31b How this money is spent   176
32   Primary symptoms found in terminal illness   194
33   QALY Language   205
34   Time trade-off for a chronic health state
     preferable to death   208
35   Classification of states of illness   212
36   Rosser's Valuation Matrix   213
37   The subjects interviewed to rank states of
     illness   214
38   Cost/QALY data adapted from Gudex (1987)   218

ACKNOWLEDGEMENTS

I am deeply grateful to all the staff at the Cancer Research Campaign Clinical Trials Centre, King's College Hospital, London, who assisted me in the preparation of this book, especially Angela McPherson, Joan Houghton and Andrea Buchanan. Thanks are also due to many other colleagues and friends for endless conversations about the measurement of quality of life, for commenting on drafts of certain chapters or providing me with helpful source material. In particular, I should like to thank Michael Baum, Andrew Clark, Patricia Day, Carol Duncan, Stephen Ebbs, Angela Hall, John Mollon, Tom Treasure, Charles Turton and Richard Vincent. Any errors contained within the book are of course entirely my responsibility.

Finally, I wish to acknowledge the immense contribution of my secretary, Ruth Sutton, who tackled the invidious task of preparing the manuscript with fortitude, skill and admirable good humour.

I should like to thank the following for permission to quote extracts from published books: The Bodley Head and William Morrow and Company Inc for *Zen and the Art of Motorcycle Maintenance* by R.M. Pirsig; International Thomson Publishing Services Ltd for *Images of Ourselves*, edited by Jo Campling, and for 'A Wish' from *Selves* by Laurence Lerner, both published by Routledge; Faber & Faber Ltd for 'Miss Gee' from *Collected Poems* by W.H. Auden; The Bodley Head and the Estate of Primo Levi for *If This is a Man* by Primo Levi, translated by Stuart Woolf; the Executors of the Virginia Woolf Estate and The Hogarth Press for 'On Being Ill' from *Collected Essays* by Virginia Woolf; Edward Arnold for *The*

Management of Terminal Disease by Dame Cicely Saunders; Tavistock Publications and Dr Colin Murray Parkes for his Foreword to *On Death and Dying* by Elisabeth Kübler Ross; David Higham Associates Limited for 'Do not go gentle into that good night' from *The Poems* by Dylan Thomas, published by Dent; J.M. Dent for 'A Song of Living' by Amelia Josephine Burr, from *Poetry Please*; Lion Publishing for *The 20th Century Plague* by C. Collier; Chapman & Hall for *AIDS: Psychiatric and Psychological Perspectives* edited by L. Paine, published by Croom Helm.

Extracts from the Authorised King James Version of the Bible, the rights of which are vested in the Crown in perpetuity within the United Kingdom, are reproduced by permission of Eyre & Spottiswoode Publishers, Her Majesty's Printers, London. The extract taken from *Why I Am Not a Christian* by Bertrand Russell is reproduced by kind permission of Unwin Hyman Ltd. The excerpt from *Illness as Metaphor* by Susan Sontag, copyright © 1977, 1978, by Susan Sontag, published London, 1979, by Allen Lane, is reproduced by permission of Penguin Books Ltd and Farrar, Straus & Giroux, Inc. The excerpt from *The Second Coming* by Walker Percy, copyright © 1980 by Walker Percy, published by Martin Secker & Warburg and Farrar, Straus & Giroux, Inc., is reprinted by permission of McIntosh and Otis, Inc.

I am grateful to the following for allowing me to reproduce copyright tables and figures: The American Medical Association and Dr Sidney Katz for 'The Katz Index of Activities of Daily Living', copyright 1963, American Medical Association; Pergamon Press plc and Dr W.O. Spitzer for 'The Spitzer Quality of Life Index'; The Macmillan Press Ltd and Dr Peter Selby for 'The Selby Linear Analogue Self-assessment Scale'; Elsevier Science Publishers BV and Dr R. Melzack for 'The McGill Pain Questionnaire'; Academic Press London Ltd and Dr H. Schipper for 'The Functional Living Index: Cancer'; Croom Helm and Professor J. McEwen for 'The Nottingham Health Profile'; NFER/Nelson for the 'General Health Questionnaire' and the 'Profile of Mood States'; Clinical Psychometric Research, Inc and Dr L.R. Derogatis for 'Psychological Adjustment to Illness Scale'; J.P. Lippincott Co. and Dr M. Bergner for the 'Sickness Impact Profile'; The

EORTC Data Centre, Brussels, and Dr N.K. Aaronson for 'The EORTC Lung Cancer Module'; Baillière Tindall for 'Psychosocial Problems of Cancer Patients'; the American Heart Association and Dr M.-L. Niemi for 'Quality of Life after Stroke'; American Congress of Rehabilitation Medicine and Dr A.M. Jette for 'Functional Status Index'; Edward Arnold and Dr A.H. Pattie for 'Clifton Assessment Procedures for the Elderly'; Pergamon Press plc and Professor G. Torrance for 'Time Trade-Off for a Chronic Health State Preference to Death'; Elsevier Science Publishers BV and Dr P. Kind for two tables from the Rosser and Kind valuation matrix; Dr Claire Gudex for 'Cost/QALY data'. The 'Health Assessment Questionnaire', courtesy of Dr J.F. Fries, and the 'Arthritis Impact Measurement Scale', courtesy of Professor R.F. Meenan, are reprinted from *Arthritis and Rheumatism Journal* 23 (2): 137–52, copyright 1980, by permission of the American College of Rheumatology.

PREFACE

Seven years ago one of the best friends I ever had developed leukaemia. Without treatment she would certainly have succumbed quickly but there was a chance, albeit a slim one, that chemotherapy and a bone marrow transplant might cure her. She was in her early thirties, happily married with two young children, and willing to try anything which might help her to live a little longer. The therapy was unsuccessful, but worse still were the toxic, unpleasant side-effects of treatment. The hair loss, nausea, vomiting, skin reactions and infections that she endured were awful to witness. Trying to communicate with a person isolated and sick in a specially constructed room for immunosuppressed patients is not easy. One sits behind a plastic window unable to touch or offer any comfort. Thus one of the most intelligent, sensitive, warm and generous-hearted people I have ever known spent some of her final weeks cut off from physical contact with most of her family and friends. I am still haunted by the last conversation we had, when she asked why I had not tried to dissuade her from a therapy with poor chances of survival, but a high chance of destroying the quality of whatever life she had left. I do not know the answer to that question, but acknowledgement of her courage and recollection of the physical and mental anguish that she suffered provided the primary impetus for writing this book.

INTRODUCTION

The advancements made in medical science this century have completely transformed the practice of medicine. In 1900 doctors still had very little to offer even those patients suffering from fairly common diseases: medicine was much more an art than a science. Hung on the walls of our prestigious medical colleges are oil paintings of eminent physicians who would determine the diagnosis and then deliver the prognosis with dramatic and flamboyant style to their impressed, awestruck students. There were, however, few really efficacious treatments available for the unfortunate patient. The primary role of most doctors was therefore to provide comfort. This was achieved by developing a good bedside manner, adopting a somewhat paternalistic responsibility for the patient, proffering a diagnosis and monitoring the progress of the disease. With limited surgical techniques and few of the pharmacological products which we take for granted nowadays, such as antibiotics or insulin, the doctor assumed a priest-like role in contrast to the scientific or highly technical role displayed by many specialists today.

We have developed impressive diagnostic procedures, therapies, drugs and surgical techniques which have revolutionised the management of hitherto fatal conditions. There are countless examples of the success of this medical revolution. The lives of premature babies and those with congenital malformations can often be saved. We have eradicated smallpox, and in most of the western world have either contained or developed treatments for other diseases which used to ravage mankind, such as cholera, typhoid, yellow fever, leprosy and malaria. Diseased organs such as hearts, lungs, livers and kidneys can be replaced. Modern surgery can restore sight, reconstruct shattered limbs and repair or replace worn-out hips, valves, veins and arteries. The lives of severely brain-damaged individuals can be maintained almost indefinitely with artificial ventilation, and modern resuscitative drugs and equipment permit us to restart the hearts of cardiac patients who have 'died'. Doctors possess a vast armoury of powerful cytotoxic drugs which provide curative treatment for certain cancers, and many previously fatal infections can be effectively treated with the large number of modern antibiotics available. Life itself can be created in the laboratory test-tube with the techniques of *in vitro* fertilisation, and recent research into genetic engineering promises the possibility of reducing many congenital abnormalities or heritable diseases. Since the turn of the century medicine and improvements in diet, housing and other social changes have dramatically increased the life expectancy of individuals.

Unfortunately, the impressive list of advancements in the *science* of medicine appears to have led to a decline in the *art* of medicine. Patients complain increasingly that 'high-tech' medicine dehumanises them. In the eternal quest for a new and better treatment for every known ailment, we have started to forget the other important needs of sick people, in particular, their emotional well-being. There are actually states of life that are worse than death and remarkably few people accept the 'life-at-any-cost' philosophy assumed by many doctors. We must consider both the quality as well as the quantity of life for any individual who requires medical treatment. This must involve moral and philosophical judgements as well as purely scientific ones, and many doctors feel ill-equipped emotionally or have been inadequately trained to deal with such issues. The attitude is therefore encouraged that it is better by far to do what is technically and financially possible from a therapeutic point of view and leave any further considerations for the social scientists and others to sort out later! The necessity to address more thoroughly the measurement of quality of life becomes more urgent as the possibilities for maintaining life increase.

1 PHILOSOPHICAL ISSUES

The world can function without it (quality), but life would be so dull as to be hardly worth living. In fact, it would not be worth living. The term worth is a Quality term. Life would just be living without any values or purpose at all.   Pirsig, 1974

What is Quality of Life?
Conceptually, quality of life is a somewhat vague term. We are all capable of expressing ideas and opinions as to what the phrase 'quality of life' means for us as individuals at any given time. Trying to define it explicitly, in a fashion which would permit objective measurement, is another matter. The nine-teenth-century philosopher and scientist, Lord Kelvin, once said:

When you can measure what you are speaking of and express it in terms of numbers, you know something about it. When you cannot express it in terms of numbers, your knowledge of it is of a meagre kind.

The politician, the philosopher, the priest, the psychologist, the poet, the physician and the patient would all offer rather different definitions of what constitutes quality of life, and few of these definitions would suggest an obvious congruent or consistent method of measurement. Maybe for some of the people just mentioned the scientific measurement of quality of life is irrelevant anyway. However, as far as quality of life in medicine is concerned, we do need to specify more precisely what we mean by the term and we must develop appropriate methodology to measure quality of life accurately.

We are rapidly approaching an ethically challenging period

in modern medicine. Technology can provide us with the ability to prolong and sustain life in states of disease and disability which previously would have been fatal. Whether the mere preservation of life is worthwhile in terms of its quality for the individual or in terms of its monetary value to society, however, is a contentious issue, which will be discussed later in Chapter 9.

In this opening chapter I wish to explore in more general terms the various ways of defining quality of life, drawing on literary and philosophical as well as scientific sources. My primary reason for adopting a rather broad exploration of the dimensions of life which contribute to its quality is recognition that certain aspects are, at the moment, immeasurable but nevertheless important. Man does not inhabit a social vacuum; thus, failure to make some attempt to set those aspects of quality of life that we can measure in a wider framework will be a futile exercise. To discuss only the measurable components would be analogous to the old joke about the drunk looking for his lost keys under a lamp post, although he had dropped them elsewhere, because the light was better under the lamp!

The phrase 'quality of life' has meant different things at different periods during this century. It entered the vocabulary of the United States towards the end of the Second World War and implied the 'good life', or material affluence evidenced by possession of cars, houses and other consumer goods such as household appliances. Spare time and spare money for leisure activities and holidays also became part of the equation. The report by the Commission on National Goals, set up by President Eisenhower in 1960, widened the range of items constituting quality of life to include education, health and welfare, economic and industrial growth and the defence of the 'free' world. Ebbs et al. (1989) claim that the major political and social upheavals of the late 'sixties, which can be seen particularly in its pop music, fashions and writings, revealed a switch of emphasis from a materialistic view of quality of life towards 'personal freedom, leisure, emotion, enjoyment, simplicity and personal caring'.

Despite the appeal of material possessions, one of the primary requisites to the enjoyment of a high quality of life is good health. Indeed, good health is such an important and desired state of being that Rokeach (1973), in a study which examined the most valued end states of existence, removed health as an option for rank ordering, since every single subject valued it higher than any of the other options.

The 1970s onwards saw a heightening of interest in the quality of life during illness and its treatment. Concurrent with technological advances, patients started to demand that their doctors took a more holistic view of medical problems. This approach is reflected in the constitution of the World Health Organisation, which states that health is 'physical, mental and social well-being and not merely the absence of disease or infirmity'. By implication, this definition suggests that illness compromises not only the biological integrity of man, but also his psychological, social and economic well-being.

Thus quality of life is a multi-faceted phenomenon and any measures taken during treatment purporting to improve the quality of life must address the impact that disease and its treatment is having on a variety of dimensions, not simply physical functioning. This was recognised by Herophilus in 300 BC, who commented upon the way in which physical demise rendered much of the rest of life somewhat meaningless.

To lose one's health renders science null, art inglorious, strength effortless, wealth useless and eloquence powerless.
Quoted by Sextus Empiricus in *Adversus Ethicus*, XI.50.

Most people, therefore, would agree that quality of life is not a unitary concept, but rather a complex amalgam of satisfactory functioning in essentially four core or primary domains, listed in Table 1.

Most items contributing to well-being and life's quality can be listed within one or other of these domains and there is obviously considerable overlap. As a psychologist, I make no apology for the implied hierarchy of this classification, placing psychological status first and physical status last. Most of the traditional medical evaluations of therapy invariably reverse that order, as we shall see in Chapter 2.

TABLE 1

Quality of Life

Core Domains	Typical Items
1 Psychological	—depression —anxiety —adjustment to illness
2 Social	—personal and sexual relationships —engagement in social and leisure activities
3 Occupational	—ability and desire to carry out paid employment —ability to cope with household duties
4 Physical	—pain —mobility —sleep —appetite and nausea —sexual functioning

THE PSYCHOLOGICAL DOMAIN

Anxiety and Depression

'A merry heart doeth good like a medicine'

Proverbs, 22

Patients suffering from crippling depression and anxiety are unable to enjoy, or function adequately in, any of the other areas thought to contribute to life's quality.

Plato recognised this and the importance of treating the whole patient, mind as well as body:

As one must not try to cure the eyes without the head or the head without the body, similarly (one must not try to cure) the body without the psyche.

Socrates in Charmides. Quoted by Greer (1987)

It is important, therefore, that due regard be paid to ensuring that any psychological problems experienced by patients are recognised and, furthermore, treated promptly and appropriately. For some patients this might mean counselling or cognitive behaviour therapy, whilst others with severe depression and/or anxiety might benefit from some short-term pharmacological intervention.

The basic rationale underpinning counselling and cognitive behaviour therapy, both of which attempt to help patients restructure their thinking and thereby their feelings and ability to cope with anxiety and depression, can be seen in the writings of the stoic philosophers such as Epictetus.

Men are disturbed not by things, but by the view which they take of them.   *The Enchiridion* (first century AD)

This approach to thinking and feeling was echoed centuries later by Shakespeare:

There is nothing either good or bad, but thinking makes it so.   *Hamlet*, Act II, Sc. ii, l. 255

Not only can cognitive therapy usefully combat anxiety and depression, it can also help the patient adjust to illness more satisfactorily.

Adjustment to Illness

One of the reasons why human beings are such successful members of the animal kingdom is their ability to adapt, adjust and cope with life in a wide range of habitats, climates and seemingly hostile environments. Survival in these situations is often dependent on necessary equipment, such as oxygen supplies and light for life underwater, or underground, and appropriate clothing for life in arctic or tropical zones. Likewise emotional survival or a healthy psychological status can only be maintained in those individuals who are capable of adapting and adjusting to the trials and tribulations of life. Some people are unable to face the fact of ill-health and its treatment unless they have access to a great deal of support from health professionals, family and friends. Others seem to be able to summon up enormous resources of fortitude, courage, dignity and even joyfulness, despite disability, pain and the threat of death. The poet Sir John Davies reflects this sentiment, that 'the Soul springs not from the Body's humours', in his poem *Nosce Teipsum*:

If she were but the body's quality
Then would she be with it sick, maim'd and blind,
But we perceive, where these privations be,
A healthy, perfect and sharp-sighted mind.

The philosophy to which I subscribe, suggesting that good psychological functioning permits an individual to adapt and cope with an awesome array of physical and social assaults, can also be seen in the testimonies of survivors of the Nazi concentration camps. Frankl, for example, witnessed first hand the mental and physical privations of the camps and later developed a branch of psychotherapy (logotherapy) based on his experiences. He is fond of a quotation from Nietzsche which aptly highlights the importance of having some purpose for living: 'He who has a why to live can bear with any how.'

A similar theme is found in Primo Levi's moving and horrific accounts of Auschwitz. In the following passage, he demonstrates the ability of some individuals to find something positive to sustain them even when close to starvation and working in freezing, wet conditions with inadequate clothing:

It is lucky that it is not windy today. Strange how in some way one always has the impression of being fortunate, how some chance happening, perhaps infinitesimal, stops us crossing the threshold of despair and allows us to live. It is raining, but it is not windy. Or else, it is raining and it is also windy: but you know that this evening it is your turn for the supplement of soup, so that even today you find the strength to reach the evening. Or it is raining, windy and you have the usual hunger, and then you think that if you really had to, if you really felt nothing in your heart but suffering and tedium—as sometimes happens, when you really seem to lie on the bottom—well, even in that case, at any moment you want you could always go and touch the electric-wire fence, or throw yourself under the shunting trains, and then it would stop raining.

Levi, 1987

Healthy psychological functioning, that is freedom from anxiety or depression and the ability to adapt and adjust to different illness states, is crucial for the maintenance of a good quality of life. It may even sustain life.

> Care to our coffin adds a nail, no doubt,
> And every grin so merry draws one out.
>
> John Wolcot (Peter Pindar), *Expostulatory Odes* XV

THE SOCIAL DOMAIN

Social Relationships

Chronic ill-health is depressing, and the chronic sick frequently express fears that friends and lovers will abandon them.

> Be glad and your friends are many,
> Be sad, and you lose them all,
> There are none to decline your nectared wine,
> But alone you must drink life's gall.
>
> Ella Wheeler Wilcox, *Solitude*

A sad example of this problem can be seen in the following passage. It is from a conversation that I had in 1982 with a young man of 26 with multiple sclerosis. For the first four years following the diagnosis, his problems with vision and mobility had been fairly minor. A further exacerbation of the illness in the six months before our conversation, however, had left him with an obvious speech impairment and difficulty with walking.

I know that my friends are starting to find it difficult to take me out with them. I mean, it was all right for a while, bit of a novelty really, their chance to show what good mates they were. But I think that they're fed up with it all now. It's not as though I've broken my leg playing football and a few weeks in plaster and I'll be all right. I'm going to get worse and I can feel them drifting away. I don't blame them, really. I'd probably be the same. I mean, cramps the style a bit, doesn't it, trying to chat up the women in the pub when you've got a bloke in a wheelchair with you, who spills his drink, talks like he's drunk before he's even had a few pints. I don't even drink much beer now, as I'm frightened I'll piss myself. They're embarrassed and so am I. I used to be one of the lads, but I'm not now. I don't want them to just feel sorry for me

and take me out, but I don't want to be on my own on a
Saturday night either.   GS (1982)

There is some evidence from anthropological work that this
fear of abandonment during illness is not entirely misplaced,
nor is it always demonstrative of neurosis or paranoia.
Avoidance behaviour might well have served a vital function
throughout evolution for both animals and prehistoric man. In
the absence of any means of treating disease, avoiding the sick
or abandoning them would have been an important adaptive
behaviour. Such seemingly callous, selfish acts would have
limited the exposure of healthy members of the species to
contagious infections, thus promoting their survival (Foster
and Anderson, 1978). This behaviour is still apparent in non-
human primates such as chimpanzees and was common in
biblical times, if one remembers the way in which lepers were
made outcasts. As we shall see later, in the chapters on cancer
and AIDS, sufferers from these two diseases are often worried
that they will be subjected to abandonment, this very primitive
form of 'quarantine'. There can be few occasions in life when
the love and support of friends and family is more important
than when ill, especially if the sufferer has chronic, progressive
or terminal disease, hence the aphorism: 'A faithful friend is
the medicine of life.' (*Ecclesiasticus* 6:16)

Sexual Relationships
Major sexual problems can occur as a result of both physical
impairment and emotional traumas. Anxiety that any attempts
at sexual activity will fail or be rejected by a partner can have a
devastating impact on an individual's quality of life. Even if full
sexual intercourse is no longer possible, most people still enjoy
the warmth and satisfaction of affectionate cuddling, kissing
and intimate non-coital caressing. The stress and strain of
attempting to maintain a sexual relationship following paralysis
can be seen in this poignant description given by a young
woman, permanently injured in a car crash:

In intimate relationships there is also that first moment
when the mechanics of your bladder management are
revealed. This is the major test. How will he react to a
mature woman who wears plastic knickers, pads and

requires help when going to the loo? . . . Even when sexually aroused, the spontaneity can soon disappear when your partner has to help empty your bladder and carefully clean and position you.   Campling (1981)

For most individuals, sick or well, touching is a basic human need, confirming that they are loved and wanted. Those people denied physical intimacy and tenderness, due to mutilating surgery and chronic or life-threatening disease, are extremely vulnerable to depression. Likewise the partner of the patient might need support and help to explore new ways of expressing love and gaining sexual gratification.

Most patients experiencing acute forms of ill-health find that the resultant physical immobility, pain, and sometimes hospitalisation pose an obvious restriction on their social and occupational activities. This is not invariably true, however, as some short-term illnesses or operative procedures can lead to a great show of love, attention and concern from family members, friends and work colleagues. Indeed, the rituals of visits, get-well cards, flowers, fruit and other gifts can serve an immensely satisfying function. They provide the 'victim' with an opportunity to see how many people 'care'. This can sometimes have the unfortunate effect of making certain insecure people adopt a 'sick-role' as an almost permanent state, especially if it is the only mechanism available to them for gaining any attention. It is not uncommon to find individuals who 'enjoy' ill-health.

Stable support from family and friends, together with the ability to participate in social activities, are immensely important contributory factors to quality of life.

THE OCCUPATIONAL DOMAIN
Part of an individual's concept of self is derived from the various social roles he or she engages in, such as work. A great deal of personal gratification is obtained through the achievement, the social recognition and the social interactions provided at and by work. Any forced retirement due to ill-health severely threatens self-image, self-worth and self-respect, which can produce considerable psychological distress. With his usual insight, Galen, writing in the second century

AD, noted that 'Employment is nature's physician, and is essential to human happiness.'

Good occupational functioning not only means the ability to carry out paid employment, but also includes the ability to cope with household duties. Dependency on others for the routine necessities of life, such as shopping, cooking and cleaning, can for many people cause a fundamental role-loss with a concomitant loss of self-esteem. It is worth remembering, however, that employment is not always particularly satisfying for some individuals. Even apparently interesting, well-remunerated occupations can be so stressful or time-consuming that they detract from life's quality by intruding on other areas. Ruskin identified three prerequisites for fulfilling and satisfying work:

> Now in order that people may be happy in their work, these three things are needed: They must be fit for it; they must not do too much of it; and they must have a sense of success in it.   John Ruskin, *Pre-Raphaelitism*

THE PHYSICAL DOMAIN

> An ounce of illness is felt more than an hundredweight of health.   Old Dutch Proverb

One curious feature about good health is the fact that it is noticed more by its absence than by its presence. Many writers have described their increased pleasure and appreciation of life following a serious illness. This is more than just relief at having survived, it suggests that insight or perception of health is only possible if we have experienced the loss of it. We seem to adapt to the fact of being healthy in much the same way as we quickly adapt to a constantly ticking clock. After a while we cease to hear or notice it, but if the rhythm of the tick changes, or the clock stops, our senses alert us to attend to this change. It is *change* in our environment or within ourselves that has biological significance, demanding attention, rather than steady state or homeostasis. The emotional significance or enhanced insight and perception of well-being following illness is succinctly captured in the following lines from Laurence Lerner's poem, *A Wish*:

Only ill-health, recurring, inevitable,
Can teach the taste of what it is to be well.

The relative importance of the different items found under the physical domain heading varies with the actual disease and, of course, the stage of the disease, so I will not discuss them in detail. Physical problems will be addressed later in the appropriate chapters dealing with specific diseases or stages in the life-cycle, but one area worthy of a brief mention now is that of pain.

Pain

'The art of life is the art of avoiding pain,' said Thomas Jefferson in a letter to Maria Cosway, dated 12th October, 1786.

Avoidance of pain is one of man's most basic drives and one of the primary reasons for seeking medical help. Chronic pain severely restricts a person's ability to function and enjoy life and poses considerable psychological, social and economic stresses. Although we all know personally what pain feels like for us, it is phenomenally difficult to explain or describe adequately the various qualities of sensory and affective experiences categorised broadly as pain. Virginia Woolf, in an essay entitled 'On Being Ill', captured the problem succinctly when she wrote:

The merest schoolgirl, when she falls in love, has Shakespeare and Keats to speak for her, but let a sufferer try to describe a pain in his head to a doctor and language at once runs dry.

Pain is rarely a simple sensation produced by a specific stimulus, and perception of pain is not always proportional to the stimulus. Pain is a very individual, subjective experience, ameliorated or enhanced by such things as culture, conditioning, attention and emotional state.

Historically, pain has been viewed within various spiritual and religious frameworks. Seeing pain as God's punishment for sin, some divine retribution for the sufferer's past misdemeanours, is not uncommon. I well remember a Catholic nun, working with me on a maternity ward, saying that the excessive pain being experienced by a 15-year-old girl during labour was God's punishment for her sin and that no extra analgesia should be given! Even the word pain is derived from the Latin 'poena', meaning punishment.

In the writings of Aristotle we find the notion that the experience of pain is the opposite of the experience of pleasure. Pain, however, seems quantitatively as well as qualitatively different from pleasure. Hence the old proverb, 'An hour of pain is as long as a day of pleasure.'

This is also reflected in one of Edmund Burke's essays:

> The torments which we may be made to suffer are much greater in their effect on the body and mind, than any pleasures which the most learned voluptuary could suggest or than the liveliest imagination, and the most sound and exquisitely sensible body could enjoy.
>
> *On the Sublime and Beautiful*, Pt. 1, Sect. VII

Despite some of the more mystical assertions that pain and suffering have ennobling consequences for individuals, intractable, chronic pain is more often a diminishing, humiliating, even frightening experience for a patient. It tends to supersede all other sensations and, according to Milton, has an evil quality about it:

> But pain is perfect miserie, the worst
> Of evils, and excessive, overturnes
> All patience.
>
> *Paradise Lost*, Book VI

Uncontrolled pain is one of the most feared consequences for patients with cancer, as we shall see in Chapter 3. Although pain in this disease usually heralds disease progression, it is important to remember that pain perception is always subjective. Pain can mask depression and can be the result of excessive anxiety. This fear of pain not only exacerbates the experience of it, but the anxiety itself can also be worse than the pain—as can be seen in the following lines from Sir Philip Sidney:

> Fear is more pain than is the pain it fears.
>
> *Arcadia*, Book V, 'Musidorus' Song'

The work of Cicely Saunders and others in the hospice movement has shown how pain can be controlled much more effectively if anxiety and fear of pain are conquered first of all.

CONCLUSION

Far too often, the successful outcome of treatment for disease has been measured in terms of the *length* of survival rather than the *quality* of that survival. This approach is neither good science nor good medicine. Failure to monitor the *quality* of life as well as the *quantity*, or limiting evaluation to only the physical dimensions, could lead to the acceptance of treatments which have a deleterious effect and to the rejection of those which have a beneficial or less harmful impact on all the items contributing to life's quality. In the words of Hubert Bland in *The Happy Moralist*:

Length must be measured by sensations, not by yards. The channel, for instance, if you are seasick, is longer than the Atlantic if you are not.

The sagacity, wit and wisdom of many different writers throughout history, provide us with useful insights into the multidimensional aspects of quality of life. Whilst their perceptions give us valuable indications as to what items we should be looking at when measuring quality of life, they do not give us any useful indicators as to *how* we can evaluate the relevant topics. In the next chapter, therefore, I shall give a critical overview of some of the different methodological approaches to the measurement of quality of life.

References

CAMPLING, J. (Ed) (1981). *Images of Ourselves*. London: Routledge & Kegan Paul, p. 17.

EBBS, S.R., FALLOWFIELD, L.J. and FRASER, S. (1989). 'The Treatment Outcomes and the Quality of Life', in Bunker, J. and Baum, M. (Eds), *Technology Assessment and Surgical Policy*. Cambridge University Press.

FOSTER, G.M. and ANDERSON, B.G. (1978). *Medical Anthropology*. New York: John Wiley & Sons.

GREER, S. (Ed) (1987). 'Psychological aspects of cancer', in *Cancer Surveys* 6(3). Oxford University Press.

LEVI, P. (1987). *If This is a Man. The Truce.* London: Abacus Books, Ch 14, p.137.

PIRSIG, R.M. (1974). *Zen and the Art of Motorcycle Maintenance.* London: The Bodley Head.

PRESIDENT'S COMMISSION ON NATIONAL GOALS (1960). *Goals for Americans.* Columbia University, The American Assembly.

ROKEACH, M. (1973). *The Nature of Human Values.* New York: Free Press/Macmillan.

WOOLF, V. (1966–7). *Collected Essays*, 4 vols. London: The Hogarth Press.

WORLD HEALTH ORGANISATION CONSTITUTION (1947). Geneva: *WHO Chron.*, 1:29.

2 METHODOLOGICAL ISSUES

As we have seen in the previous chapter, a completely satisfactory, all-inclusive definition of quality of life is extremely difficult to elucidate. Most people would agree that, as a concept, quality of life exists, although universal agreement as to *what* it is seems unlikely. The clinicians appear more inclined towards definitions in terms of physical function, whereas the psychosocial scientists describe it in terms of the complex inter-relationships between the physical, emotional and social domains. I do not feel that this necessarily suggests blinkered insensitivity on the part of the doctor. Too often social scientists feel that they alone are on the side of the angels and that they have a monopoly of concern for the total well-being of sick people. Meanwhile, the clinicians are portrayed as fighting the disease and ignoring the consequences that treatments have on patients' quality of life.

Stereotypes would not be so powerful if they did not have some element of truth: doubtless we have all met doctors who are so interested in the scientific challenge of curing disease that they become indifferent to the other needs of the unfortunate patient; likewise, there are social scientists who tend to forget that some people *are* prepared to sacrifice quality of life and accept unpleasant side-effects for the slight or unlikely chance of cure. Arguably, improvements in treating childhood leukaemia and testicular cancer, for example, would not have been realised had there not been clinicians who were prepared to give extremely toxic therapy and patients who were prepared to take part in phase I and II clinical trials of experimental treatment regimens. There are, however, many chronic diseases for which there is no surgical or medical cure, so that the aim of any therapy is to alleviate symptoms and hopefully improve function. In such situations therapeutic interventions must also improve quality of life if they are to be of any value. This can involve delicate balancing and trade-offs: sometimes improving or alleviating certain symptoms is only achievable at the cost of introducing others; thus the net benefit in quality of life terms may be quite marginal. A deeper discussion of this particular problem can be found in Chapter 5, in the sections reviewing the treatment of high blood pressure and angina. Clearly, many covariates in any given patient's world must be considered, and if possible their contribution evaluated, when the therapeutic effects on quality of life are being assessed.

I have spent some time trying to outline a reasonably comprehensive definition of what constitutes quality of life. Some doctors, research workers and others act as though merely labelling the questionnaire 'a quality of life schedule', or claiming that their study is assessing 'quality of life', bestows some magical validation properties upon the test items and investigation. Despite the seductive titles, many studies purporting to assess quality of life have chosen a ludicrously narrow definition of the concept, such as 'ability to return to full-time paid employment', or 'ability to manage household tasks'. An example of this can be found in an article entitled 'The Quality of Life after Liver Transplantation' (Starzl *et al.*, 1979). The authors looked at quality of life in 44 survivors of 139 liver transplants where survival meant life beyond one year post-transplant. Eighteen survivors died approximately two years later, usually from liver failure and/or rejection, and most of this time was spent in hospital receiving a variety of treatments. The authors conclude, however, that the 26 patients still living achieved a 'very high' degree of rehabilitation. This meant that they had returned to work, school or housework. Little is said about impairments to psychosexual life and none of this important information is quantified. Nevertheless, the concluding sentence states: 'The *complete rehabilitation* of so many patients has encouraged us to continue our efforts in this difficult field.'

In 1981 Najman and Levine published the results of a literature search done by them, investigating the assessment tools used to evaluate quality of life in a variety of studies purporting to examine the impact of medical technology on outcome. During the period spanning 1975–79 they found 23 studies, 22 of which employed some 'objective' measure of 'quality of life', and only three of these attempted any subjective assessments. Najman and Levine contrasted the sophistication of the medical technologies with the methodological inaccuracies of the work evaluating the impact of these technologies. They described the instruments used as '. . . weak, unconvincing, superficial and possibly misleading', and concluded by stating that, 'while it may be the case that some interventions do improve the quality of life, the inadequacies of the studies undertaken to date do not provide convincing support for such an argument.' So what are the methods currently available for assessing quality of life? What are their limitations? How can we choose an appropriate measure? And what direction should future research be taking in the development of tests?

There are many different approaches to the measurement of quality of life, all reflecting different theoretical traditions. The tests which I shall describe are chosen to demonstrate the wide variety of techniques currently being used. This is not meant to imply that they are necessarily the best tests available, but has much more to do with their frequency of usage in the medical literature. More information about quality of life measures specific to certain diseases or stages in the life cycle will be found in relevant later chapters.

Firstly, I need to outline the basic requirements that all tests purporting to measure quality of life should satisfy. This might assist the non-specialist reader in understanding why some seemingly good tests are actually unsound and not really valid or reliable methods of assessment. Readers with a particular interest in these important issues, who require a more detailed analysis, should look no further than the excellent papers and books by Cronbach (1960), Anastasi (1976), Nachmias (1981) and Nunnally (1978).

Basic requirements of tests and measurements

1   Reliability
One of the most important criteria for determining whether or not any given test has been constructed properly is to examine

its *reliability*. Whilst it might sound a little like stating the obvious in this particular context, reliability is really asking, 'Does this test measure accurately and consistently what it is meant to be measuring?' All sorts of chance factors in an individual's life can influence his or her score on any self-rating questionnaire; but what the test developer must be able to do is indicate how inaccurate any score is likely to be as a result of these chance factors. Sensible interpretation of test scores can only be made if something is known about the test's reliability. This is crucial when health status is changing over the course of treatment or with disease progression. If the *reliability coefficient* of a test is not known, then either an improvement or a demise in the patient's quality of life might be incorrectly attributed to the therapy being given, when in fact the change in test score was due to chance factors.

The *reliability coefficient* can be determined in a number of different ways. Traditionally, two versions of the same test are administered to the intended sample population, that is people of similar age, social characteristics, sex, or disease state. If only one form is available, the test is split into two equal parts and both parts are given to the same individuals in the target population. If two test scores are similar for the group, then it is likely that the test is consistent and reliable. This technique is known as *split-test reliability*. Perfect reliability would produce a correlation coefficient of 1.00, but one would expect to find coefficients of approximately 0.90 for most good tests. To measure *test-retest reliability*, our sample population of people is given the same test on two occasions and the correlation coefficient between both scores is derived. Whilst this is theoretically simple, there are pitfalls. Of primary importance is the timing between administrations of the test. If the time difference is too short, respondents might well recall their previous answer, thus the true reliability might be over-estimated. If, on the other hand, the time interval chosen is too long, changes in bodily state, disease progression, etc., might well cause a change in test score which could lead to an underestimate of the actual reliability.

Another way of expressing how accurate or reliable test scores are is to look at the *standard error of measurement*. The complex statistical and logical bases for this measurement are not appropriate to set out in a book such as this, but the essential principles are easy to understand. The standard error provides an estimate of the range of variation in a patient's score if he or she were repeatedly to take the same test on an infinite number of occasions. Thus it is possible to compute the 'zonal' range of inaccuracy on either side of an obtained score. This is potentially very important if, for example, treatments are going to be either continued or withdrawn on the basis of some threshold score on a quality of life instrument.

In common parlance, the word 'reliable' has connotations with such things as 'worthwhile', 'good' and 'trustworthy', so it is important that clinicians, researchers and others do understand what test reliability means. A reliable test might not be a 'good' test, since merely stating that a test measures *something* reliably tells us little unless we know what that *something* is! More important than test reliability, therefore, is test *validity*.

2 *Validity*

If test developers have done their job properly, they will be able to give information about their instrument's validity. This refers to the extent to which a test measures what it purports to measure. As with reliability, this seems a fairly obvious and necessary criterion to satisfy before using any 'quality of life' instrument with patients, but it is frequently violated or ignored. This might be due to the fact that validity is more difficult to assess than reliability and frequently involves quite extensive analysis of many different correlations between measures. There are four primary types of validity: face, content, criterion and construct validity.

Face validity examines whether or not the items within the test appear, on a subjective evaluation, to be asking questions relevant to the purpose of the test. For example, in a new test measuring memory function following brain injury, one might expect to find questions concerning the name of the current prime minister or the capital of France; but such items would probably lack validity in a quality of life scale. (On the other hand, the impact that a particular prime minister or a trip to Paris has on the quality of life of an individual, might well be relevant!)

Content validity is basically looking at how comprehensive a coverage of the important constructs of interest has been made. For example, in a quality of life schedule designed for use with patients who had been receiving chemotherapy for cancer, one might expect to find many items dealing with the potential side-effects of treatment. Likewise, a measure designed to assess the benefits of coronary artery bypass surgery for heart disease might need to look at items such as return to paid employment or leisure activities following relief of chest pain and breathlessness. The traditional way of establishing which items should be included in an instrument to ensure good content validity is to interview typical patients and ask them very open-ended questions to determine the important areas of concern. The problems most frequently cited by patients should then be incorporated into the questionnaire or interview schedule.

It is necessary to study the *criterion validity* if a test is designed as a predictive measure. This is done by correlating the test item scores with some previously validated criterion measure and establishing a validity coefficient. It is most unusual for these coefficients to be anywhere near as high as those demanded for reliability. Validity coefficients as low as 0.30 are often quite acceptable. One might predict, for example, that high anxiety pre-operatively would correlate with excessive demands for analgesics for pain relief post-operatively. Thus, if the object of the study was to use a psychological test to screen patients who might find their anxiety alleviated by good counselling, it would first be necessary to establish the criterion validity of the test—that is, do highly anxious people, according to the new measure, require more pain relief than those not anxious?

Another form of validity which is performed less frequently is *construct validity*. Here the measure being validated, commonly a theme, domain or construct, is tested to see if it relates to certain other constructs within the test in various hypothesised ways. This is achieved by examining the ability of the construct to discriminate between two groups of people known to differ in some particular way. For example, a construct of 'non-compliance' with diet and drugs in a study of diabetic patients should discriminate between those patients whose diabetes was well-controlled and those who had frequent hypo or hyper glycaemic attacks. It is possible, however, that the hypothesis being tested is unsound. Failure to discriminate between well-controlled and uncontrolled diabetic patients could be due to factors other than the compliance/non-compliance construct, for example the failure of the physician to prescribe the correct units of insulin, the refractory nature of the disease, or faulty scales when measuring food. One of the statistical methods used to test construct validity is *factor analysis*. In a quality of life measure such as the Rotterdam Symptom Checklist, which will be described in detail later, two constructs or subscales are identified following factor analysis: *physical problems*, which include such things as hair loss, vomiting and diarrhoea; and *psychological problems*, which include items such as worry or feeling desperate about the future. Factor analysis used to be quite a lengthy and complex process, but computer programs have given people less excuse for not analysing the hypothesised clusters of items supposedly making up the constructs within any new test.

Related to both content and construct validity is *specificity*, which is the ability of any quality of life measure to identify correctly different populations of patients. One would expect a test with good specificity to be able to discriminate between those individuals experiencing a good quality of life and those experiencing a poor one. Taking the example of a questionnaire assessing psychological disturbances such as anxiety, specificity would be calculated from the following:

$$\frac{\text{number of true cases of anxiety}}{\text{number of true non-cases of anxiety and false positive cases}}$$

This computation yields a percentage score for specificity. The *sensitivity* score of an instrument tells us about the accuracy of the measure in picking up changes in a patient's quality of life, due to such things as disease progression or remission and psychological status. Sensitivity is calculated from the following:

$$\frac{\text{number of true cases}}{\text{number of true cases plus false negative scores}}$$

In the previous section I mentioned that reliability was less important than validity, but that statement needs some further qualification. If the test is unreliable, then validity will also be low. Any valid test will by definition be reliable. However, an instrument can be extremely reliable but not valid. If I were to be given a test of 'basic linguistic ability in foreign languages' for example, which contained items such as, what are the words or phrases for 'hello', 'thank-you' and 'goodbye' in Dutch, Chinese and Urdu, I would definitely fail. This test, however, would be extremely reliable, that is I would achieve the same score on repeated occasions (with a correlation coefficient of 1.00!) and the split-test reliability would also be 1.00. This reliable 'test' would, however, be invalid as it violates almost every validity requirement. If the same test asked for translations in a wider range of languages, such as French, German, Italian, Greek and Spanish, and added extra basic words such as colour, numbers, days of the week and months, thus improving the face and content validity for a test purporting to assess 'basic linguistic ability in foreign languages', my scores would improve slightly; and when compared with another group of 39-year-old female academics, might well demonstrate that my skills in that domain were slightly below average.

This might seem a faintly ludicrous example, but there are 'quality of life' measures analogous to my 'linguistic ability' test which 'reliably' measure only a limited aspect of quality of life. Those dealing almost solely with physical functioning might well suggest that quality of life is very good. I hope that I have by now argued the case for considering more than physical functioning in such instruments. Following surgery for bowel cancer, a man might well have a perfectly functioning colostomy and no sign of metastatic spread of the disease. This would produce both a high and reliable score on health performance scales such as the Karnofsky (1947). That same patient, might, however, be deeply anxious about recurrent disease, severely depressed about impotence or loss of attractiveness to his sexual partner; he might also have stopped working due to fears of odour or leakage from the bag, and given up a sporting activity such as swimming. It hardly requires a test to show that such a person has suffered a considerable decline in life's quality. A performance index might be reliable; it might also be valid as far as physical functioning is concerned, but these indices are clearly invalid measures of quality of life.

3   Norms and Standardisation
In evaluating tests and interpreting their scores, we also have to consider, alongside reliability and validity, the manner in which the various scores are being expressed. A numerical score tells us very little about an individual's quality of life, unless we have further information about the scores which most people of a similar age, sex, social class, educational background or disease state would have in similar circumstances. In *standardised* tests, scores are derived or transformed in a manner which permits the individual scores to be compared with group norms. There is a variety of methods to make raw scores more meaningful and the most appropriate method is really dependent on the way in which the test has been designed. (See, for example, Seashore, 1955.)

When dealing with global scores from tests purporting to measure quality of life, it is very important to know more about the mean and standard deviations from it, in order to analyse the data satisfactorily. Transformations of raw scores into standard-deviation units allow psychologists or anyone else who knows anything about normal distribution curves to see immediately how far above or below average an individual lies. This enables comparisons to be made which are not possible with the raw scores alone.

*   *   *

Reliability, validity and standardisation are just a few of the issues that test developers must consider. It is also important for test *users* to have some grasp of the complexity of these points, to enable them to assess the relative merits of available instruments before launching off to develop one of their own.

WHICH TEST?
Having examined some of the methodology of test design, this is probably an appropriate time to discuss some of the constraints which might influence the choice of quality of life

questionnaires. Table 2 provides a summary of the areas to consider before choosing a quality of life measure.

TABLE 2

THINGS TO CONSIDER WHEN CHOOSING A TEST

1 Is it valid and reliable?
2 Are norms available?
3 Is it suitable for target population?
4 Are questions easy to read and understand?
5 Is scoring easy or complex?
6 Is the layout of the questionnaire clear?
7 What is the format of the questions?
8 Is it comprehensive but as brief as possible?
9 Does it ask socially loaded questions?
10 Who will complete questions—doctor or patient?

Is it suitable for the target population?

It is most unlikely that any one quality of life measure will be equally suitable for all the different age groups and medical specialities requiring assessment. Some tests, for example the Sickness Impact Profile (SIP) or the Psychosocial Adjustment to Illness Scale (PAIS), have a large number of questions relating to sexual activity and interest. This might well offend some populations of patients or be quite insensitive and irrelevant to others. On the other hand, ignoring such items as sex in studies of patients who have undergone gynaecological or genito-urinary and bowel surgery, might result in a very incomplete assessment of the impact of treatment.

Are the questions easy to read and understand?

The level of literacy in a general population of patients is usually much lower than most research workers realise. If patients cannot read and understand the language used in the questionnaire, then compliance will be low or respondents will get others to fill in the forms for them. Many 'off the shelf' quality of life schedules were developed in America, and American is a surprisingly difficult language for some English-speaking people to understand. If the age range of the patients being studied is high, then questionnaires may need to have large print. For example, the 28-item General Health Questionnaire (GHQ) has much larger printing than the 60 or 30 item GHQ.

Is scoring easy or complex?

Quality of life measures for routine use by clinicians, perhaps as screening devices in their out-patient clinics, must be quick and easy to score. Those measures used as part of a research protocol can probably afford to be more complex, especially if there are research assistants, statisticians and others to assist with data analysis. If scoring takes too long, however, the measures will never gain acceptance amongst busy clinicians. Further discussion of the problems encountered when analysing quality of life data can be found at the end of this chapter.

Is the layout of the questionnaire clear?

If the layout of the questionnaire is complex or unclear, the quality of the data declines. Not only will patients miss out important sections, but it also complicates the analysis of the questionnaire.

In what format are the questions and responses?

Most of the common quality of life schedules in use are self-assessment questionnaires employing linear analogue or categorical scaling. *Visual analogue scales* employ lines, usually ten centimetres long, with stops at each end. The length of the line represents the continuum of an emotional or physical experience, such as anxiety or pain, and the patient is asked to mark the line at the point which corresponds to his or her perception of that experience. The ends of the lines denote the extremes, from best to worst, of the experience being considered. Some patients require help in grasping the concept, but it is a technique that has been used successfully with five-year-olds (Scott *et al.*, 1977). Although easy for patients to complete, visual analogue scales are rather difficult to score.

Categorical scales are usually quick and simple to complete and score, as they are pre-coded. Patients are instructed to tick a labelled box corresponding to their perception of the item in question. For example, 'Do you feel anxious?' might have four possible response categories, such as 'very much', 'moderately', 'somewhat' or 'not at all'. These are then given a numerical score from nought to three or one to four. There have been many arguments about the most appropriate number of categories. Too many categories can produce unreliability as patients might find it difficult to discriminate between shades of meaning; too few categories might not provide an appropriate range of responses (Fayers and Jones, 1983). If the numerical scores from items of subsets within a rating scale are added together to form a single score, this is known as a Likert scale. These are fairly easy to analyse and generally have good reliability coefficients.

Guttman Scales are another type of rating scale sometimes seen in quality of life tools. In these, patients make a 'yes or no' response to various items grouped together in degrees of severity or difficulty. These responses can then be scored from nought to three or one to four.

Other quality of life measurements used include categorical rating scales, indices or profiles filled in by the physician (observer ratings) and interview schedules which require trained interviewers. Examples of all these will be discussed in more detail later.

Is it comprehensive but as brief as possible?
The instruments currently available for quality of life measurement vary in dimensional range and depth. Consequently, to fulfil all the requirements of a thorough assessment, several questionnaires may be necessary. The number of measures needed is dependent on the aims of the person conducting the assessment. A research protocol for quality of life evaluation in a clinical trial might require a more extensive test than a screening questionnaire in an out-patient clinic. A basic heuristic to follow is that the briefer the questionnaire, the better the compliance. A balance always has to be struck between overloading patients with forms to complete in order to achieve a comprehensive cover, and sacrificing some depth of questioning so as to ensure compliance and improve the accuracy of responses. This consideration is particularly important when making repeated assessments of physically sick people who may resent the added burden of excessive form-filling. The over-zealous researcher can reduce the

quality of the information gained by striving for too much. Lengthy questionnaires increase the likelihood of patients agreeing with all statements, irrespective of content.

What is the time-frame of the questionnaire?

Some quality of life measures have variable time-frames from a few days to a few weeks, whilst others give no indication at all of the time-frame. Whoever administers the questionnaires must ensure that respondents are aware of the period being considered, otherwise the risk of error increases. It is advisable to have as short a time-frame as possible to improve the accuracy of recall. Trying to remember how much pain or anxiety, or how much coughing, one has experienced over the preceding month is much more difficult than recall of the same items over the preceding three days.

Does it ask socially loaded questions?

It requires considerable skill to frame questions in such a way so as to minimise implied value judgements or prevent patients from giving the socially desirable responses. In some cultures and amongst patients of different sex, age or social class, there might be a variety of reasons for either under- or over-reporting symptoms. Patients are sometimes reluctant to admit to their care-givers that treatments are making them feel much worse. Others may feel that being a 'good' patient will make their doctors and nurses work harder at curing them and so they, too, will under-report symptoms (Luce and Dawson, 1975). Some males find it difficult to admit to pain or to emotional distress. It is particularly difficult to overcome the bias of socially desirable responding in interview schedules when the interviewer is someone intimately involved with the patient's care, such as a doctor or nurse. The presence of a friend or relative is also likely to reduce the reliability of responses to certain questions, especially those concerned with coping, relationships, sex and pain.

Who will complete the questionnaire—patient or doctor?

Many clinicians favour rating scales that they themselves can fill in, on the grounds that they can use clinical judgement and be more objective than patients. Correlation coefficients for measures made by patients and their doctors are invariably low, however, suggesting that doctors cannot accurately determine their patients' mood states or problems. A recent study by Slevin and colleagues (1988) showed that not only was there poor agreement between doctors and their patients about quality of life, but that there was also wide variability in scores between different doctors and other health professionals. Slevin concludes that '. . . if measurement of a patient's quality of life is required, it should be done by the patients themselves and not their doctors and nurses.'

WELL-KNOWN QUALITY OF LIFE MEASURES IN MEDICINE

Performance indices and observation scales completed by the physician

The Karnofsky Performance Index (KPS)

This performance index is one of the most frequently cited 'quality of life' measures found in the medical literature. A review of papers under the heading 'quality of life' in *Index Medicus* by Grieco and Long (1984) showed that it was used more than any other instrument. Frequency of usage is, however, no indication of appropriateness. Karnofsky and Burchenal actually developed their performance scale as a means of determining nursing requirements on a ward; they claimed that with other subjective and objective measures it provided '. . . a measure of the usefulness of the patient or the burden that he represents to his family or society'. The KPS is a serviceable method of determining physical functioning and it has been shown to correlate well with survival, but it remains a crude method for evaluating quality of life. The primary difficulties with the KPS are that it is filled in by the physician, and that it makes no assessment of a patient's psychosocial status. Table 3 shows the categories of functioning contained within the scale. Ratings are made by the clinician from 100 per cent to zero. One hundred per cent represents normal functioning with no evidence of disease, and zero represents the terminal point, in other words death. Clark and Fallowfield

(1986), in a review of quality of life measurements, point out some absurdities of the scale, in particular the assumption that a patient with a lowish score due to immobility is considered to have a poor quality of life and that a patient with a higher score necessarily has a better quality of life. They cite the example of an incontinent paraplegic or wheelchair-bound multiple-sclerosis victim, who would score only 40 per cent on the KPS. Even if the patient was well-adjusted to the fact of his or her illness, had good social support and experienced rich and happy relationships with others, he or she would, using a KPS scale, have a poor quality of life score. Contrast this situation with that of a breast cancer patient who might have a score of 80 per cent. She might well be so emotionally crippled by depressive illness—which the scale does not assess—that her loss of self-esteem, interest in social functioning, concentration levels and sexual activities meant that quality of life was rather poor, although the KPS score would suggest the reverse to be true.

TABLE 3

The Karnofsky Performance Index

Description	Scale %
Normal, no complaints	100
Able to carry on normal activities; minor signs or symptoms of disease	90
Normal activity with effort	80
Cares for self. Unable to carry on normal activity or to do active work	70
Requires occasional assistance but able to care for most of his needs	60
Requires considerable assistance and frequent medical care	50
Disabled; requires special care and assistance	40
Severely disabled; hospitalisation indicated although death not imminent	30
Very sick. Hospitalisation necessary. Active supportive treatment necessary	20
Moribund	10
Dead	0

An important criticism, common to all observation scales, is the fact that assessment involves an entirely subjective evaluation made by the clinician. Bias inevitably arises and there are studies showing quite unacceptable variability between raters; for example, one study by Hutchinson *et al.* (1979) reported inter-rater agreement to be less than 34 per cent. Correlation coefficients are also poor when patients' self-ratings are compared with those of other health professionals. Clinicians often underestimate the dysfunction and impact that illness exerts on well-being. I have already mentioned the Slevin study (1988) which showed the poor correlation between doctors and their patients. This was also found in the United States of America by Nelson and colleagues (1983). Grieco and Long (1984) have attempted to revise the KPS and, using trained observers, they managed to improve such things as inter-rater reliability and to show correlations between KPS scores and other quality of life measures.

The KPS was never designed as a quality of life measure, yet this simple scale has been used more widely and for longer than any other. This prominence rests on the test's longevity and its usefulness as a crude predictor of survival rather than on any demonstrable soundness as an appropriate quality of life measure. The World Health Organisation (WHO) has produced an alternative but similar scale to the KPS. This WHO scale is shown in Table 4 and consists of a physician-completed, five-point physical performance scale. It is simple to use and interpret, but shares many of the limitations of the KPS; in particular the narrow range of assessment emphasising physical functioning and neglecting psychosocial variables.

The Katz Index of Activities of Daily Living (1963)
Another performance index which has stood the test of time, despite some reservations about its validity as a quality of life measure, is the Activities of Daily Living Index (ADL) developed in 1963 by Katz. Its primary use was in the assessment of functional status of elderly patients in long-term care settings. Nurses or clinicians rate patients on six items: bathing, dressing, toileting, mobility, continence and feeding.

TABLE 4

World Health Organisation Performance Status

Grade	Performance status
0	Able to carry out all normal activity without restriction.
1	Restricted in physically strenuous activity but ambulatory, but able to carry out light work.
2	Ambulatory and capable of all self-care but unable to carry out any work; up and about more than 50% of waking hours.
3	Capable of only limited self-care; confined to bed or chair more than 50% of waking hours.
4	Completely disabled; cannot carry on any self-care; totally confined to bed or chair.

Patients are rated as either dependent or independent for each item and then graded from A to G according to these judgements. Table 5 shows the definitions of dependence or independence and the grades used in the ADL. As with the KPS, high grades on the ADL do correlate well with survival (Katz *et al.*, 1970), and it has been shown to be of prognostic value in determining the long-term course of adaptation in stroke victims or patients with fractures of the hip. A major problem limiting the scale's usefulness in studies is its inability to discriminate well between differences in functioning at the upper end of the scale. As the reader will see in Chapter 8, approximately 80 per cent of elderly people do not experience functional limitations and the ADL would give all these people the same score. Clearly, other indices would be necessary if the object of the study was to evaluate quality of life.

In summary, this scale has good validity and reliability and it has been helpful in measuring the functional status of elderly institutionalised patients; but the application of the scale in general population studies of quality of life is not appropriate. There have been many adaptations of the ADL: in particular, those scales designed for use with arthritic patients such as the Arthritic Impact Measurement Scale (AIMS). These will be described in detail in Chapter 6.

TABLE 5

SOME DEFINITIONS AND GRADES FOR THE KATZ INDEX OF ACTIVITIES OF DAILY LIVING

Index of Independence in Activities of Daily Living

The index of independence in activities of daily living is based on an evaluation of the functional independence or dependence of patients in bathing, dressing, going to the toilet, transferring, continence, and feeding. Specific definitions of functional independence and dependence appear below the index.

A　　　Independent in feeding, continence, transferring, going to toilet, and bathing.

B　　　Independent in all but one of these functions.

C　　　Independent in all but bathing, and one additional function.

D　　　Independent in all but bathing, dressing, and one additional function.

E　　　Independent in all but bathing, dressing, going to toilet, and one additional function.

F　　　Independent in all but bathing, dressing, going to toilet, transferring, and one additional function.

G　　　Dependent in all six functions.

Other　Dependent in at least two function, but not classifiable as C, D, E, or F.

Independence means without supervision, direction, or active personal assistance, except as specifically noted below. This is based on actual status and not on ability. A patient who refuses to perform a function is considered as not performing the function, even though he is deemed able.

eg Bathing (sponge, shower or tub)

Independent: assistance only in bathing a single part (as back or disabled extremity) or bathes self completely

Dependent: assistance in bathing more than one part of body: assistance in getting in or out of tub or does not bathe self

The Spitzer Quality of Life Index

An interesting physician-scored observation scale is the QL Index developed by Spitzer *et al.* in 1981, for use with cancer patients. These authors established clearly defined criteria when developing their test. It had to be quick to complete (less than one minute); simple to administer, score and analyse; and able to address a more comprehensive range of quality of life dimensions than simple physical functioning. Following a considerable amount of field-work using cancer patients, people suffering from other chronic diseases, lay people, doctors, nurses and social workers, Spitzer *et al.* identified five key areas to evaluate. These areas can be seen in Table 6. Activity, daily living, perception of health, social support and outlook on life are all rated on a three-point scale from nought to two, giving a maximum score of ten.

The authors have reported good inter-rater reliability between physicians and, more importantly, good correlations between patients' self-ratings and those of their clinicians. It has been validated on patient populations in both Australia and Canada and discriminates well between patients with different illnesses and at different stages of disease. One of the scale's limitations is the fact that it gives equal weighting to all items contained within the index, which seems unrealistic. Furthermore, there are not enough items within each key area to allow sufficient specificity of problems. Clark and Fallowfield (1986) highlight the difficulty this might pose for rating in, for example, the daily living section where self-reliance in eating, washing, toileting, dressing, using public transport or driving own car are all lumped together. It is possible that the personal care items could be achieved with the patient housebound and quite unable to use transport.

The primary strength of this scale has to be its simplicity and speed. I mentioned at the beginning of this chapter the difficulty of coercing busy clinicians and nurses to use quality of life measures if they are too complex or take too long to complete. Despite its limitations, the QL Index seems worth further research and can be recommended for use with cancer patients. Although originally developed for use by physicians, the index can also be used in self-assessment by patients.

TABLE 6

Spitzer's Quality of Life Index

Score each heading 2, 1 or 0 according to your recent assessment of the patient.

ACTIVITY

During the week, the patient
- has been working or studying full time, or nearly so, in usual occupation: or managing own household: or participating in unpaid or voluntary activities, whether retired or not.................2
- has been working or studying in usual occupation or managing own household or participating in unpaid or voluntary activities: but requiring major assistance or a significant reduction in hours worked or a sheltered situation or was on sick leave...............1
- has not been working or studying in any capacity and not managing own household...............0

DAILY LIVING

During the last week, the patient
- has been self-reliant in eating, washing, toileting and dressing; using public transport or driving own car...............2
- has been requiring assistance (another person or special equipment) for daily activities and transport but performing light tasks...............1
- has not been managing personal or light tasks and/or not leaving own home or institution at all...............0

HEALTH

During the last week, the patient
- has been appearing ro feel well or reporting feeling 'great' most of the time...............2
- has been lacking energy or not feeling entirely 'up to par' more than just occasionally...............1
- has been feeling very ill or 'lousy', seeming weak and washed out most of the time or was unconscious...............0

SUPPORT

During the last week
- the patient has been having good relationships with others and receiving strong support from at least one family member and/or friend...............2
- support received or perceived has been limited from family and friends and/or by the patient's condition...............1
- support from family and friends occurred infrequently or only when absolutely necessary or patient was unconscious...............0

OUTLOOK

During the past week the patient
- has usually been appearing calm and positive in outlook, accepting and in control of personal circumstances including surroundings...............2
- has sometimes been troubled because not fully in control of personal circumstances or has been having periods of obvious anxiety or depression...............1
- has been seriously confused or very frightened or consistently anxious and depressed or unconscious...............0

Self-assessment Questionnaires and Tests

VISUAL ANALOGUE SCALES (VAS)

Linear analogue self-assessment (LASA)
Priestman and Baum (1976) developed their 25-item test to measure the impact that breast cancer and its treatment had on the quality of life. Table 7 provides an example of the four different categories in which patients produced self-ratings. The Priestman and Baum LASA probes four main areas: the symptoms and effects of disease and treatment, such as pain and nausea; psychological problems such as anxiety and depression; physical indices such as ability to perform housework; and finally items concerned with personal relationships. The test has been used successfully in studies comparing quality of life of patients receiving either endocrine or cytotoxic therapy for breast cancer (Baum *et al.*, 1980) and appears to have good sensitivity and reliability. There are some worrying criticisms of the test, however, which are difficulties for all measures that employ VAS methods: the scales are time-consuming to score; the scores may not always relate well to the experience being considered; the theoretically fine discrimination which is possible might not be 'real'; and finally,

TABLE 7

Some Items from the LASA (Priestman and Baum)

DIFFICULTY WITH SLEEP
    Most nights ———————————————⊣ Never
FEELING OF WELL BEING
    Very bad ———————————————⊣ Very good
RELATIONSHIP WITH PARTNER
    Impossible ———————————————⊣ Excellent
RELATIONSHIP WITH OTHER PEOPLE
    Impossible ———————————————⊣ Excellent
SEXUAL RELATIONSHIPS
    Total loss ———————————————⊣ Better than ever
DECISION MAKING
    Impossible ———————————————⊣ Excellent
ABILITY TO PERFORM HOUSEWORK
    Impossible ———————————————⊣ Better than ever

there is a lack of any weighting of the variables being measured. It is not always true that patients exhibiting equal changes in scores over a period of time reveal the same evidence of either improvement or deterioration. The clinical significance of changes in scores is not always obvious.

Selby's LASA

Another linear analogue self-assessment scale designed for use specifically in clinical trials of cancer treatment is the Selby LASA shown in Table 8. This scale contains 32 items, most of which were derived from the Sickness Impact Profile to be described later. Early work has been encouraging, showing good reliability coefficients and satisfactory discrimination between clinically distinct groups of patients (Selby *et al.*, 1984). The author and his colleagues are still developing the test, however, and are attempting to address the problem I highlighted above when discussing the Priestman and Baum LASA, namely that of weighting different items within the test and providing test norms. If these difficulties are overcome, the test looks promising for use with cancer patients.

The McGill/Melzack Pain Questionnaire (MPQ)

Without doubt, chronic unremitting pain imposes a severe deleterious effect on quality of life. Consequently, a satisfactory pain inventory, despite its apparent specificity, does constitute an important element of quality of life assessment. In 1971 Melzack and Torgerson developed a systematic and objective measure of pain, known as the McGill Pain Questionnaire (MPQ), and it is the most widely used pain inventory in both clinical practice and research. The MPQ comprises groups of adjectives, some of which are shown in Table 9, and these rank values are scored to provide a pain rating index. The tool has been shown to be highly reliable and valid (Melzack, 1975), and can be used successfully with patients as young as 12 years. Many questionnaires employing visual analogue scales have been developed using items adapted from the MPQ to assess pain.

TABLE 8

Part of Selby's LASA

Please score how *you feel* each of these aspects
of your life was
affected by *the state of your health*,
during *today* (24 hrs)

19   *Depression*
extremely ———————————————————— not depressed
depressed   at all

20   *Appearance of your body*
extremely ———————————————————— completely
dissatisfied   satisfactory
(because of the   for me at
state of my health,   my age
 disease or treatment)

21   *Family relationships and marriage/cohabitation*
extremely ———————————————————— normal family
bad relationships   life for me
because of the state
of my health

22   *Housework*
no housework ——————————————————— normal house-
because of the   hold duties
state of my health   for me

23   *Eating* (increased or decreased)
COMPLETE (a) or (b)
 (a)
not eating ————————————————————— normal eating
                                                                                       for me

 (b)
greatly ———————————————————————— normal eating
increased eating   for me

TABLE 9

McGill Pain Questionnaire

What does pain feel like?
Tell which words best describe your present pain
Use only a single word in each appropriate group the one that applies best
Indicate answer with (√)

1
1. flickering
2. quivering
3. pulsing
4. throbbing
5. beating
6. pounding

2
1. jumping
2. flashing
3. shooting

3
1. pricking
2. boring
3. drilling
4. stabbing
5. lancinating

4
1. sharp
2. cutting
3. lacerating

5
1. pinching
2. pressing
3. gnawing
4. cramping
5. crushing

6
1. tugging
2. pulling
3. wrenching

7
1. hot
2. burning
3. scalding
4. searing

8
1. tingling
2. itchy
3. smarting
4. stinging

9
1. dull
2. sore
3. hurting
4. aching
5. heavy

10
1. tender
2. taut
3. rasping
4. splitting

11
1. tiring
2. exhausting

12
1. sickening
2. suffocating

13
1. fearful
2. frightful
3. terrifying

14
1. punishing
2. gruelling
3. cruel
4. vicious
5. killing

15
1. wretched
2. blinding

16
1. annoying
2. troublesome
3. miserable
4. intense
5. unbearable

17
1. spreading
2. radiating
3. penetrating
4. piercing

18
1. tight
2. numb
3. drawing
4. squeezing
5. tearing

19
1. cool
2. cold
3. freezing

20
1. nagging
2. nauseating
3. agonising
4. dreadful
5. torturing

The Functional Living Index: Cancer (FLIC)

This scale, developed by Schipper and colleagues (1984) in Canada, is a good example of a *graded* linear analogue scale (see Table 10). It contains 22 items which were produced after a considerable and lengthy validation process, including the establishment of sub-scales following factor analyses (factor analysis is a statistical method establishing the relationship between items in a test). Some workers have argued against providing numbered categories along linear analogue scales; for example, Scott and Huskisson point out that when patients were asked to rate pain along a 20-point scale, number ten and 15 appeared to be particularly 'favoured', showing that respondents might have marked their favourite numbers. One of the doyens of test design, Guilford (1954), stated that lines of such scales should be solid, with no breaks or divisions, to ensure optimal use of the technique. Notwithstanding these comments, Schipper *et al.* appear to have researched their instrument well, although they have yet to produce data showing satisfactory correlations with other instruments, and doubts remain as to whether or not it has sufficient items for each dimension to detect accurately significant changes in quality of life over a period of time.

Nottingham Health Profile (NHP)

This health profile was developed by Hunt and McEwen (1980) as a survey tool, but has been used increasingly in this country to evaluate the outcome of medical interventions (Hunt, McEwen and McKenna, 1985). The authors of the NHP have conducted an enormous volume of research to refine their instrument and to produce evidence that it is both reliable and valid. The NHP is divided into two parts. Part 1 (see Table 11a) consists of 38 statements which can be sub-divided under six problem areas: energy, pain, emotional reactions, sleep, social isolation and physical mobility. Part 2 (shown in Table 11b) has seven statements concerning the areas of daily life which are often affected by ill-health: paid employment, jobs around the house, social life, personal relationships, sex life, hobbies and interests, and holidays. Respondents are required to answer 'yes' or 'no' to statements such as 'things are getting me down'. Each statement has a

TABLE 10

ITEMS FROM MANITOBA CANCER TREATMENT and RESEARCH FOUNDATION FUNCTIONAL INDEX: CANCER (FLIC)

Date

1. Most people experience some feelings of depression at times. Rate how often you feel these feelings.

1	2	3	4	5	6	7
Never						Continually

2. How well are you coping with your everyday stress?

1	2	3	4	5	6	7
Not well						Very well

3. How much time do you spend thinking about your illness?

1	2	3	4	5	6	7
Constantly						Never

4. Rate your ability to maintain your usual recreation or leisure activities.

1	2	3	4	5	6	7
Able						Unable

5. Has nausea affected your daily functioning?

1	2	3	4	5	6	7
Not at all						A great deal

6. How well do you feel today?

1	2	3	4	5	6	7
Extremely poor						Extremely well

7. Do you feel well enough to make a meal or do minor household repairs today?

1	2	3	4	5	6	7
Very able						Not able

8. Rate the degree to which your cancer has imposed a hardship on those closest to you in the past 2 weeks.

1	2	3	4	5	6	7
No hardship						Tremendous hardship

9. Rate how often you feel discouraged about your life.

1	2	3	4	5	6	7
Always						Never

10. Rate your satisfaction with your work and your jobs around the house in the past month.

1	2	3	4	5	6	7
Very dissatisfied						Very satisfied

11. How uncomfortable do you feel today?

1	2	3	4	5	6	7
Not at all						Very uncomfortable

PLEASE INDICATE WITH + YOUR RATING

weighting attached to it reflecting the perceived relative importance or severity of the item. High scores are associated with severe problems, thus the maximum score in both Part 1 and Part 2 of the test is 100.

Not only does the NHP discriminate well between fit and physically sick people (the authors tested it on firemen and mine-rescue workers), but it is sensitive enough to detect changes throughout the different trimesters of pregnancy. One of the difficulties with using it as a quality of life measure is the problem that it only looks at negative aspects of health, making it impossible for patients to indicate well-being accurately. Zero scores do not necessarily reflect the absence of problems and it might be difficult for the profile to detect relatively small but nevertheless significant areas of distress. However, this well-researched instrument is worth considering as a quality of life measure in view of its acceptability, cheapness and easy scoring.

The General Health Questionnaire (GHQ)

There are three different versions of Goldberg's GHQ, containing 28, 30 or 60 items (Goldberg, 1972). Only the 28-item test will be described here, as this is the one usually chosen by clinicians as a quality of life measure. The GHQ-28 has four sub-scales assessing depression, anxiety, social functioning and physical symptoms. Patients underline the response that matches most closely their perception of how they have been feeling about each of the 28 item statements, as shown in Table 12. Scoring is quick and simple and it can be done in two different ways: either employing a Likert-type score of zero to three, or using a bimodal response scale with 'less' or 'no more' than usual scoring zero and 'rather' or 'much more' than usual scoring one. This particular method gets around the problem of 'end-users' or 'middle users', that is those patients who always respond at the extremes of scales or always use the middle options. The GHQ has good reliability and has been satisfactorily validated against the Clinical Interview Schedule. It also performs well against other psychiatric screening tests. As the test has been used in many different clinical settings and in community studies involving large numbers of people, it is an instrument well worth considering as part of a quality of life

TABLE 11a

Nottingham Health Profile
(Some items from Part 1)

Listed below are some problems people may have in their daily life.

Look down the list and put a tick in the box under 'yes' for any problem you have at the moment.

Tick the box under 'no' for any problem you do not have.

Please answer every question. If you are not sure whether to say yes or no, tick whichever answer you think is more true at the moment.

	YES	NO
I'm tired all the time	☐	☐
I have pain at night	☐	☐
Things are getting me down	☐	☐

	YES	NO
I have unbearable pain	☐	☐
I take tablets to help me sleep	☐	☐
I've forgotten what it's like to enjoy myself	☐	☐

	YES	NO
I'm feeling on edge	☐	☐
I find it painful to change position	☐	☐
I feel lonely	☐	☐

	YES	NO
I can only walk about indoors	☐	☐
I find it hard to bend	☐	☐
Everything is an effort	☐	☐

TABLE 11b

Nottingham Health Profile
(Part 2)

Now we would like you to think about the activities in your life which may be affected by health problems.

In the list below, tick 'yes' for each activity in your life which is being affected by your state of health. Tick 'no' for each activity which is not being affected, or which does not apply to you.

YES NO

Is your present state of health causing problems with your . . .

JOB OF WORK
(That is, paid employment) ☐ ☐

LOOKING AFTER THE HOME
(Examples: cleaning and cooking, repairs, odd jobs round the home, etc.) ☐ ☐

SOCIAL LIFE
(Examples: going out, seeing friends, going to the pub, etc.) ☐ ☐

HOME LIFE
(That is: relationships with other people in your home) ☐ ☐

SEX LIFE ☐ ☐

INTERESTS AND HOBBIES
(Examples: sports, arts and crafts, do-it-yourself, etc.) ☐ ☐

HOLIDAYS
(Examples: summer or winter holidays, weekends away, etc.) ☐ ☐

TABLE 12

THE GENERAL HEALTH QUESTIONNAIRE

GHQ 28
David Goldberg
(Part A)

Please read this carefully.

We should like to know if you have had any medical complaints and how your health has been in general, *over the past few weeks*. Please answer ALL the questions on the following pages simply by underlining the answer which you think most nearly applies to you. Remember that we want to know about present and recent complaints, not those that you had in the past.

It is important that you try to answer ALL questions.

Thank you very much for your co-operation.

Have you recently

A1 — been feeling perfectly well and in good health?	Better than usual	Same as usual	Worse than usual	Much worse than usual
A2 — been feeling in need of a good tonic?	Not at all	No more than usual	Rather more than usual	Much more than usual
A3 — been feeling run down and out of sorts?	Not at all	No more than usual	Rather more than usual	Much more than usual
A4 — felt that you are ill?	Not at all	No more than usual	Rather more than usual	Much more than usual
A5 — been getting any pains in your head?	Not at all	No more than usual	Rather more than usual	Much more than usual
A6 — been getting a feeling of tightness or pressure in your head?	Not at all	No more than usual	Rather more than usual	Much more than usual
A7 — been having hot or cold spells?	Not at all	No more than usual	Rather more than usual	Much more than usual

assessment. Its limitation is the fact that it assesses primarily physical functioning and psychological status, so other quality of life dimensions would need to be determined using other questionnaires.

The Rotterdam Symptom Checklist (RSCL)

This instrument was introduced by De Haes *et al.* (1983) to measure the toxicity and impact that treatment for cancer was having on psychosocial functioning or quality of life. Respondents rate different items on a four-point scale by ticking a box opposite the reply which comes closest to how they have been feeling over the previous three days. There are approximately 30 items which can be divided into two primary subscales measuring physical and psychosocial dimensions. Additional items for assessment of treatment, or illness-related variables, are often included; for example, Table 13 shows a version of the RSCL used with patients who have breast cancer. Items concerned with body image have been added. Work is still in progress to establish population norms, but there are data emerging that show good sensitivity and specificity for the psychological items on the scale and these have been validated against trained interviewer ratings. The test is extremely easy to understand and patients find it quite acceptable (Fallowfield *et al.*, 1986). Furthermore, it is simple to administer and only takes five to ten minutes to complete. Scoring is straightforward and easy to compute. Hopefully the authors of the RSCL will be able to provide us with a handbook and norms so that the test can be incorporated into all clinical trial protocols and recommended for routine use by clinicians to assess quality of life.

Psychological Adjustment to Illness Scale (PAIS)

One of the most impressive tests developed in recent years, which could be used to evaluate quality of life in a variety of patient populations, is the PAIS (Morrow *et al.*, 1978). Its authors, Morrow, Chiarello and Derogatis, are eminent research workers, especially in the field of cancer. Their experience gained from studying the psychosocial impact of ill-health has resulted in an extremely comprehensive instrument. It was originally a semi-structured interview, administered by

TABLE 13

Items in The Rotterdam Symptom Checklist (RSCL)

Name_____ Title_____ Date of birth_____
Date_____Occupation_____Hospital_____

In this questionnaire you will be asked about your symptoms.
Read each item and place a firm tick in the box opposite the
reply which comes closest to how you have been feeling during
the last three days.

SECTION I

1. Lack of appetite
   Not at all
   A little
   Somewhat
   Very much

2. Irritability
   Not at all
   A little
   Somewhat
   Very much

3. Worry about my health
   Not at all
   A little
   Somewhat
   Very much

4. Tiredness
   Not at all
   A little
   Somewhat
   Very much

5. Worrying
   Not at all
   A little
   Somewhat
   Very much

6. Sore muscles
   Not at all
   A little
   Somewhat
   Very much

7. Depressed
   Not at all
   A little
   Somewhat
   Very much

8. Lack of energy
   Not at all
   A little
   Somewhat
   Very much

9. Pain
   Not at all
   A little
   Somewhat
   Very much

10. Nervousness
    Not at all
    A little
    Somewhat
    Very much

11. Nausea
    Not at all
    A little
    Somewhat
    Very much

12. Feel desperate about the future
    Not at all
    A little
    Somewhat
    Very much

13. Difficulty in falling asleep
    Not at all
    A little
    Somewhat
    Very much

14. Headache
    Not at all
    A little
    Somewhat
    Very much

15. Vomiting
    Not at all
    A little
    Somewhat
    Very much

16. Feeling self-conscious
    Not at all
    A little
    Somewhat
    Very much

17. Dizziness
    Not at all
    A little
    Somewhat
    Very much

18. Lack of sexual interest
    Not at all
    A little
    Somewhat
    Very much

19. Feel lonely
    Not at all
    A little
    Somewhat
    Very much

20. Dissatisfied with my appearance
    Not at all
    A little
    Somewhat
    Very much

21. Feel tense
    Not at all
    A little
    Somewhat
    Very much

trained doctors, nurses, psychologists or social workers, but is now available in a self-report questionnaire. The test has 45 questions looking at a patient's global adjustment to illness in seven important areas affecting quality of life:

1   *health care orientation*—their attitudes towards and expectations concerning physicians and treatments;
2   *vocational environment*—satisfaction with job performance and adjustment to work;
3   *domestic environment*—the impact of illness on family finances and communication;
4   *sexual relationships*—effect illness has had on frequency, satisfaction and pleasure from sexual activity;
5   *extended family relationships*—problems with extended family members since illness;
6   *social environment*—the maintenance of interest in social activities;
7   *psychological distress*—anxiety, depression, etc.

You might recall the core domains, listed in Table 1, which I suggested any adequate quality of life scale should address; the PAIS appears to cover them all well. The cost of this comprehensive coverage, however, is the complexity of scoring the test and the time that it takes patients to complete (approximately 30 minutes). Ratings for each question are made on a four-point scale, examples of which can be seen in Table 14. These scores are then converted to standardised T-scores found in tables in the handbook, providing a PAIS total score which can then be compared with published norms. The wealth of research done by the authors means that, unlike many other measures, there are norms available for a variety of patient populations such as cardiac, renal and cancer patients. The test has good reliability coefficients and correlates well with other tests measuring psychological dimensions. Adjustment to the fact of illness and its treatment, especially in chronic diseases, exerts an important influence on quality of life which the PAIS measures extremely well.

TABLE 14

Some items from Section VI of PAIS

SECTION VI—SOCIAL ENVIRONMENT

(1) INDIVIDUAL LEISURE INTEREST

Are you still as interested in your leisure time activities and hobbies as you were prior to your illness (i.e. watching TV, sewing, bicycling, etc.)?

[   ] 0 = same level of interest as previously
[   ] 1 = slightly less interest than before
[   ] 2 = significantly less interest than before
[   ] 3 = little or no interest remaining

(2) INDIVIDUAL LEISURE ACTIVITIES

How about actual participation? Are you still actively involved in doing those activities?

[   ] 0 = participation remains unchanged
[   ] 1 = participation reduced slightly
[   ] 2 = participation reduced significantly
[   ] 3 = little or no participation at present

(3) FAMILY LEISURE INTEREST

Are you as interested in leisure time activities with your family (i.e. playing cards and games, taking trips, going swimming, etc.) as you were prior to your illness?

[   ] 0 = same level of interest as previously
[   ] 1 = slightly less interest than before
[   ] 2 = significantly less interest than before
[   ] 3 = little or no interest remaining

The Sickness Impact Profile (SIP)

Developed by Bergner *et al.* in 1976, this is one of the most widely used and best known quality of life questionnaires. It comprises 136 items, divided into 12 categories, derived from an original pool of 312 statements concerning the impact of sickness on behavioural function (Bergner *et al.*, 1981). The selected 136 statements can be divided into independent categories: those concerned with physical function and those to do with psychosocial functioning—see Table 15. Patients respond with a 'yes' or 'no' to each statement. The scale values for each SIP statement were determined from judgements made by 25 health care professionals, patients and lay people who used a 15-point scale of dysfunction from maximal to minimal. All statements endorsed by the patient completing the SIP have their scale values added up to yield a percentage overall score. Depending on the purpose in using the SIP, either an overall score or scores for the two principal dimensions can be computed. Validity and reliability for the SIP are impressive and its authors have conducted a substantial body of research to update and improve the questionnaire. Few of the quality of life measures currently available have undergone such extensive work on validation and reliability. Thus it has been the measure of choice in a large number of different studies looking at evaluations of treatment following hip replacement, in hyperthyroidism, arthritis and obstructive pulmonary disease. However, such a comprehensive measure, together with its methodological refinements, has made it rather cumbersome and time-consuming. Repeated measures on very sick people might represent an intolerable burden and few clinicians would have time for the detailed analysis demanded. These limitations make it unacceptable for routine use, but it is an important measure to consider in clinical trial protocols.

*   *   *

Very few of the currently available psychometric tools purporting to measure quality of life achieve more than a cursory assessment of an individual's psychological status. Similarly, clinicians rarely make adequate judgements about the impact that treatment has on a patient's psychological functioning—indeed, studies have shown that they often fail to detect clear evidence of psychiatric morbidity amongst their patients. For example, Maguire *et al.* (1978) claim that 80 per cent of clinically depressed or anxious patients post-mastectomy go unrecognised as such by their surgeons. If patients are overwhelmed by depression or suffering from crippling anxiety they will experience a very poor quality of life. Such

TABLE 15

Some of the Sickness Impact Profile Categories and Selected Items

Dimension	Category Items Describing Behaviour Related to:	Selected Items
Independent categories	Sleep and rest	I sit during much of the day
		I sleep or nap during the day
	Eating	I am eating no food at all, nutrition is taken through tubes or intravenous fluids
		I am eating special or different food
I. Physical	Ambulation	I walk shorter distances or stop to rest often
		I do not walk at all
II. Psychosocial	Body care and movement	I do not bathe myself at all, but am bathed by someone else
		I am very clumsy in body movements
	Social interaction	I am doing fewer social activities with groups of people
		I isolate myself as much as I can from the rest of the family
	Emotional behaviour	I laugh or cry suddenly I act irritable and impatient with myself, for example, talk badly about myself, swear at myself, blame myself for things that happen

psychological problems disrupt social relationships, work and leisure activities and enjoyment of life as profoundly as those provoked by physical problems. It is important, therefore, that quality of life questionnaires which lack a reasonable assessment of psychological distress should be supplemented by a scale to measure mood states.

SCALES TO ASSESS MOOD STATE

The Profile of Mood States (POMS)

This was originally developed in 1979 by Pollock *et al.* and later refined for marketing by McNair *et al.* (1981). It provides an assessment of an individual's current emotional state by asking subjects to rate how applicable 65 different mood descriptions are to them. Subjects are given semantic differentials, i.e. phrases such as 'not at all' through to 'extremely', which permit them to express the degree to which items such as 'sad' apply. There are six different subscales on the POMS: tension, depression, anger, vigour, fatigue and confusion (see Table 16 for examples). Work has shown good specificity on the POMS subscales.

The Hospital Anxiety and Depression Scale (HAD)

This was developed by Zigmond and Snaith (1983) specifically for use with physically sick populations. It has two subscales— anxiety and depression—and does not include items of a somatic nature, for example tiredness, which could be caused by physical disease as much as mood disturbance. The test consists of 14 items, seven for each subscale, and patients rate items on a four-point scale as shown in Table 17. One further advantage of the HAD is that it is extremely easy and quick to administer, complete and score. (Few patients require more than two minutes to complete it and scoring takes about the same time.) Validation against the Clinical Interview Schedule shows that it has satisfactory sensitivity and specificity. Another useful aspect of the HAD concerns the fact that it has been translated into many different languages, including most European, Japanese, and some Asian languages. This, together with the test's quickness, makes it a very suitable measure to use routinely amongst hospital patients, as it can be used with multi-ethnic populations.

TABLE 16
Part of the POMS

Below is a list of words that describe feelings people have. Please read each one carefully. Then fill in ONE circle under the answer to the right which best describes HOW YOU HAVE BEEN FEELING DURING THE PAST WEEK INCLUDING TODAY.

	NOT AT ALL	A LITTLE	MODERATELY	QUITE A BIT	EXTREMELY
1. Friendly	(0)	(1)	(2)	(3)	(4)
2. Tense	(0)	(1)	(2)	(3)	(4)
3. Angry	(0)	(1)	(2)	(3)	(4)
4. Worn out	(0)	(1)	(2)	(3)	(4)
5. Unhappy	(0)	(1)	(2)	(3)	(4)
6. Clear-headed	(0)	(1)	(2)	(3)	(4)
7. Lively	(0)	(1)	(2)	(3)	(4)
8. Confused	(0)	(1)	(2)	(3)	(4)
9. Sorry for things done	(0)	(1)	(2)	(3)	(4)
10. Shaky	(0)	(1)	(2)	(3)	(4)
11. Listless	(0)	(1)	(2)	(3)	(4)
12. Peeved	(0)	(1)	(2)	(3)	(4)
13. Considerate	(0)	(1)	(2)	(3)	(4)
14. Sad	(0)	(1)	(2)	(3)	(4)
15. Active	(0)	(1)	(2)	(3)	(4)
16. On edge	(0)	(1)	(2)	(3)	(4)
17. Grouchy	(0)	(1)	(2)	(3)	(4)
18. Blue	(0)	(1)	(2)	(3)	(4)
19. Energetic	(0)	(1)	(2)	(3)	(4)
20. Panicky	(0)	(1)	(2)	(3)	(4)

	NOT AT ALL	A LITTLE	MODERATELY	QUITE A BIT	EXTREMELY
21. Hopeless	(0)	(1)	(2)	(3)	(4)
22. Relaxed	(0)	(1)	(2)	(3)	(4)
23. Unworthy	(0)	(1)	(2)	(3)	(4)
24. Spiteful	(0)	(1)	(2)	(3)	(4)
25. Sympathetic	(0)	(1)	(2)	(3)	(4)
26. Uneasy	(0)	(1)	(2)	(3)	(4)
27. Restless	(0)	(1)	(2)	(3)	(4)
28. Unable to concentrate	(0)	(1)	(2)	(3)	(4)
29. Fatigued	(0)	(1)	(2)	(3)	(4)
30. Helpful	(0)	(1)	(2)	(3)	(4)
31. Annoyed	(0)	(1)	(2)	(3)	(4)
32. Discouraged	(0)	(1)	(2)	(3)	(4)
33. Resentful	(0)	(1)	(2)	(3)	(4)
34. Nervous	(0)	(1)	(2)	(3)	(4)
35. Lonely	(0)	(1)	(2)	(3)	(4)
36. Miserable	(0)	(1)	(2)	(3)	(4)
37. Muddled	(0)	(1)	(2)	(3)	(4)
38. Cheerful	(0)	(1)	(2)	(3)	(4)
39. Bitter	(0)	(1)	(2)	(3)	(4)
40. Exhausted	(0)	(1)	(2)	(3)	(4)

TABLE 17
HAD Scale

Doctors are aware that emotions play an important part in most illnesses. If your doctor knows about these feelings he will be able to help you more.

This questionnaire is designed to help your doctor to know how you feel. Read each item and place a firm tick in the box opposite the reply which comes closest to how you have been feeling in the past week.

Don't take too long over your replies: your immediate reaction to each item will probably be more accurate than a long thought-out response.

Tick only one box in each section

I feel tense or 'wound up':
Most of the time ....
A lot of the time ....
Time to time, Occasionally ....
Not at all ....

I still enjoy the things I used to enjoy:
Definitely as much ....
Not quite so much ....
Only a little ....
Hardly at all ....

I get a sort of frightened feeling as if something awful is about to happen:
Very definitely and quite badly ....
Yes, but not too badly ....
A little, but it doesn't worry me ....
Not at all ....

I can laugh and see the funny side of things:
As much as I always could ....
Not quite so much now ....
Definitely not so much now ....
Not at all ....

Worrying thoughts go through my mind:
A great deal of the time ....
A lot of the time ....
From time to time but not too often ...
Only occasionally ....

I feel cheerful:
Not at all ....
Not often ....
Sometimes ....
Most of the time ....

I can sit at ease and feel relaxed:
Definitely ....
Usually ....
Not often ....
Not at all ....

I feel as if I am slowed down:
Nearly all the time ....
Very often ....
Sometimes ....
Not at all ....

I get a sort of frightened feeling like 'butterflies' in the stomach:
Not at all ....
Occasionally ....
Quite often ....
Very often ....

I have lost interest in my appearance:
Definitely ....
I don't take so much care as I should.....
I may not take quite as much care ....
I take just as much care as ever ....

I feel restless as if I have to be on the move:
Very much indeed ....
Quite a lot ....
Not very much ....
Not at all ....

I look forward with enjoyment to things:
As much as ever I did ....
Rather less than I used to ....
Definitely less than I used to ....
Hardly at all ....

I get sudden feelings of panic:
Very often indeed ....
Quite often ....
Not very often ....
Not at all ....

I can enjoy a good book or radio or TV programme:
Often ....
Sometimes ....
Not often ....
Very seldom ....

ANALYSIS

Adequate analysis of quality of life data is extremely important, but often neglected (Gore, 1988). The sorts of analyses applied depend to a certain extent on the use to which the information will be put. If the main purpose for asking a patient to complete a questionnaire is to use that information to tailor therapy for the individual or to apply appropriate ameliorative interventions when necessary, then problems are few. One is primarily interested in single-item scores or in looking at variables within key domains which appear to be causing difficulty. Comparison of group 'means' between patients receiving different therapies is more problematic, especially if the total numbers of patients in each group are small. One patient with an extreme score could produce a most distorted view of overall quality of life for the majority of the other patients. This demonstrates the importance of researchers understanding elementary statistics.

Another common problem concerns the pooling of all the 'scores' from different sections of a questionnaire. As Krauth (1982) has pointed out, this implies that a patient with a lowish score in one domain can be compensated in some way by high scores in other areas. A hypothetical but good illustration of this might involve a patient with multiple sclerosis experiencing further exacerbation of his or her disease leading to much reduced mobility. If this person had consequently received a specially adapted car which conveyed wheelchairs around easily, the patient's previously restricted social opportunities and independence might actually be enhanced, thus improving overall quality of life. There are absurdities, however, such as the example cited by Krauth of 'a high index of therapy success for a patient with far better interpersonal relations than before therapy, who on the other side is still producing metastases'.

CONCLUSION

When one contemplates the enormous volume of work that has been conducted by psychometricians and others in the development of quality of life measures over the past two decades, which can clearly yield vital information about the effects of disease and treatment, it seems absurd that such efforts are still derided by many medical scientists.

Do we really need to be so apologetic about our supposedly subjective data, or accepting of the frequently expressed criticism that such data are 'soft' and therefore less important or reliable than the 'hard' objective clinical data. Feinstein, in his excellent critique examining the choice of clinical variables used in research, cites ten papers to support the following passage:

> Statisticians and clinicians have been extraordinarily naïve in unquestioningly accepting as hard data the reports that are generated by pathologists and radiologists. For example, when the observer variability of pathologists has been checked for diagnosing the histopathology of cell types in cancer, the results usually show so many discrepancies and inconsistencies that the histopathologic distinctions may become impossible to interpret. Undaunted by this gross unreliability, clinicians continue to plan treatment according to cellular types, and statisticians continue to accept, code and analyse the data.

Feinstein also cites eight references to studies revealing quite 'striking' variability for both inter- and intra-observer agreement amongst radiologists. One is reminded of the Latin *duo cum facunt idem, non est idem* (when two people do the same thing, it is not the same).

Undoubtedly we still have a long way to go before a completely satisfactory, scientifically valid and acceptable measure of quality of life is developed, but there are tests currently available which can help doctors to determine the impact that their therapies are having on more than just the physical and functional aspects of their patients' lives. Failure to attempt to monitor quality of life is neither good medicine, nor is it good science.

References

ANASTASI, A. (1976). *Psychological Testing*, 4th ed. Macmillan Publishing Co. Inc., New York.

BAUM, M., PRIESTMAN, T.J., WEST, R.R. and JONES, E.M. (1980). 'A comparison of subjective responses in a trial comparing endocrine with cytotoxic treatment in advanced carcinoma of the breast', in Mouridsen, H.T. and Palshof, T. (Eds), *Breast Cancer—Experimental and Clinical Aspects*. Oxford: Pergamon Press.

BERGNER, M., BOBBITT, R.A., CARTER, W.B. and GILSON, B.S. (1981). 'The sickness impact profile: Development and final revision of a health status measure', in *Med. Care*, XIX (8), 787–805.

CLARK, A.W. and FALLOWFIELD, L.J. (1986). 'Quality of life measurements in patients with malignant disease: a review', in *JRSM*, 79: 165–9.

CRONBACH, L.J. (1960). *Essentials of Psychological Testing*, 2nd ed. New York: Harper & Row.

DE HAES, J.C.J.M., PRUYN, J.F.A. and KNIPPENBERG, F.C.E. (1983). 'Klachtenlijst voor kankerpatienten. Eerste ervaringen', in *Nederlands Tijdschrift voor de Psychologie*, 38: 403–22.

FALLOWFIELD, L.J., BAUM, M. and MAGUIRE, G.P. (1986). 'Do psychological studies upset patients?' in *JRSM*, 80: 59.

FAYERS, P.M. and JONES, D.R. (1983). 'Measuring and analysing quality of life in cancer clinical trials: a review', in *Statistics in Medicine*, 2: 429–46.

FEINSTEIN, A.R. (1977). 'Hard science, soft data, and the challenges of closing variables in research', in *Clin. Pharmacol. & Ther.*, 22: 485–98.

GOLDBERG, D. (1972). *Detection of Psychiatric Illness by Questionnaire*. Oxford University Press.

GORE, S.M. (1988). 'Integrated reporting of quality and length of life: a statistician's perspective', in *Eur. Heart J.*, 9: 228–34.

GRIECO, A. and LONG, C.J. (1984). 'Investigation of the Karnofsky Performance Status as a measure of quality of life', in *Health Psychology*, 3: 129–43.

GUILFORD, J.P. (1954). *Psychometric Methods*. New York: McGraw-Hill.

HUNT, S.M. and MCEWEN, J. (1980). 'The development of a subjective health indicator', in *Sociology of Health and Illness*, 2(3): 231–46.

HUNT, S.M., MCEWEN, J. and MCKENNA, S.P. (1985). 'Measuring health status: a new tool for clinicians and epidemiologists', in *J. Roy. Coll. Gen. Pract.*, 35: 185–8.

HUTCHINSON, T.A., BOYD, N.F. and FEINSTEIN, A.R. (1979). 'Scientific problems in clinical scales as demonstrated in the Karnofsky index of performance status', in *J. Chron. Dis.*, 32: 661–6.

KARNOFSKY, D.A. and BURCHENAL, J.H. (1949). 'The clinical evaluation of chemotherapeutic agents in cancer', in MacLeod, C.M. (Ed), *Evaluation of Chemotherapeutic Agents*. New York: Columbia University Press, pp. 191–205.

KATZ, S.T., FORD, A.B., MOSOWITZ, R.W., JACKSON, B.A. and JAFFE, M.W. (1963). 'Studies of illness in the aged', in *JAMA*, 185: 914–19.

KATZ, S.T., DOWNS, H., CASH, H. *et al.* (1970). 'Progress in the development of the index of ADL', in *The Gerontologist*, 10: 20–30.

KRAUTH, J. (1982). 'Objective measurement of the quality of life', in Baum, M. and Schuerlen, H. (Eds). *Clinical Trials in Early Breast Cancer*. Birkhauser Verlag, pp. 402–53.

LUCE, J.K. and DAWSON, J.J. (1975). 'Quality of Life', in *Seminars in Oncol.*, 2: 321–323.

MCNAIR, D.M., LORR, M. and DOPPLEMAN, L.F. (1981). *EITS manual for the profile of mood states*. San Diego: Educational and Industrial Testing Service.

MAGUIRE, G.P., LEE, E.G., BEVINGTON, D.J. *et al.* (1978). 'Psychiatric problems in the first year after mastectomy', in *BMJ*, 1: 963–5.

MELZACK, R. (1975). 'The McGill pain questionnaire: major properties and scoring methods', in *Pain*, I: 277–99.

MELZACK, R. and TORGERSON, W.S. (1971). 'On the language of pain', in *Anaesthesiology*, 34: 50–9.

MORROW, G.R., CHIARELLO, R.J. and DEROGATIS, L.R. (1978). 'A new scale for assessing patients' psychological adjustment to medical illness (PAIS)', in *Psychol. Med.*, 8: 605–10.

NACHMIAS, C. and NACHMIAS, D. (1981). *Research Methods in the Social Sciences*. London: St Martins Press.

NAJMAN, J.M. and LEVINE, S. (1981). 'Evaluating the impact of medical care and technologies on the quality of life: a review and critique', in *Soc. Sci. Med.*, 15F: 107–15.

NELSON, F., CONGER, B., DOUGLASS, R. *et al.* (1983). 'Functional health status levels of primary care patients,' *JAMA*, 249: 3331–8.

NUNNALLY, J.C. (1978). *Psychometric Theory*, 2nd ed. New York: McGraw-Hill.

POLLOCK, V., CHO, D.W., REKER, D. *et al.* (1979). 'Profile of Mood States: the factors and their physiological correlates', in *J. Nerv. Ment. Dis.*, 167: 612.

PRIESTMAN, T.J. and BAUM, M. (1976). 'Evaluation of quality of life in patients receiving treatment for advanced breast cancer', in *Lancet*, (i): 899–901.

SCHIPPER, H., CLINCH, J., MCMURRAY, A. and LEVITT, M. (1984). 'Measuring the quality of life of cancer patients. The functional living index—cancer: development and validation', in *J. Clin. Oncol.*, 2: 472–83.

SCOTT, J., ANSELL, B.M. and HUSKISSON, E.C. (1977). 'The measurement of pain in juvenile chronic polyarthritis', in *Ann. Rheum. Dis.*, 36: 186–7.

SEASHORE, H.G. (1955). 'Methods of expressing test scores', in *Psychological Corporation Test Service Bulletin*, 48: New York.

SELBY, P.J., CHAPMAN, J.A., ETAZADI AMOLI, J., DALLEY, D. and BOYD, N.C. (1984). 'The development of a method for assessing the quality of life of cancer patients', in *Br. J. Ca.*, 50: 13.

SLEVIN, M.L., PLANT, H., LYNCH, D. *et al.* (1988). 'Who should measure quality of life, the doctor or the patient?' in *Br. J. Ca.*, 57: 109–12.

SPITZER, W.O., DOBSON, A.J., HALL, J. *et al.* (1981). 'Measuring the quality of life of cancer patients', in *J. Chron. Dis.*, 34: 595–7.

STARZL, T.E., KOEP, G.P. *et al.* (1979). 'The quality of life after liver transplantation', in *Transplantation Proceedings*, XI(1); March.

WORLD HEALTH ORGANISATION (1979). *WHO handbook for reporting results of cancer treatment*. Geneva: WHO, Offset Publication No. 48.

ZIGMUND, A.S. and SNAITH, R.P. (1983). 'The Hospital Anxiety and Depression Scale', in *Acta Psychiatr. Scand.*, 67: 361–70.

3 THE QUALITY OF LIFE IN CANCER

> Nobody knows what the cause is,
> Though some pretend that they do;
> It's like some hidden assassin
> Waiting to strike at you.
>
> W.H. Auden

There are approximately a quarter of a million new cases of cancer registered each year in the United Kingdom. On the basis of these incidence rates it has been estimated that one in three people will develop cancer at some stage during their life (Cancer Research Campaign, 1988). Five cancer sites in particular account for more than half of the new cases registered: lung (17 per cent), colon and rectum (11 per cent), skin (ten per cent), breast (ten per cent) and stomach (five per cent). Table 18 shows that there is an extremely wide variation in the relative survival rates for these different cancers. Skin cancer has almost 100 per cent survival rate five years after registration, whereas only seven per cent of patients with lung cancer and four per cent of patients with pancreatic cancer are still alive after that period. Cancer currently causes the death of 160,000 people in the United Kingdom each year and is responsible for almost a quarter of all deaths.

Given these statistics, it is hardly surprising that cancer provokes more apprehension and horror than any other disease. For many patients the diagnosis is received with dread and a fear akin to being given a death sentence (McIntosh, 1974). Both the psychological and the physical consequences of the disease impose a severe threat to a patient's sense of well-being and quality of life. Not only the sufferer, but also the relatives and friends of a patient with cancer, experience a

TABLE 18

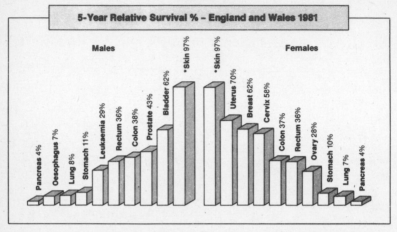

5-Year Relative Survival % – England and Wales 1981

Males

Females

Pancreas 4% · Oesophagus 7% · Lung 8% · Stomach 11% · Leukaemia 29% · Rectum 36% · Colon 38% · Prostate 43% · Bladder 62% · *Skin 97%

*Skin 97% · Uterus 70% · Breast 62% · Cervix 58% · Colon 37% · Rectum 36% · Ovary 28% · Stomach 10% · Lung 7% · Pancreas 4%

plethora of emotional difficulties. Most of this psychological trauma can be considered under two main headings:

1   the knowledge of having a life-threatening disease; and
2   a fairly uniform dread of the necessary treatments and their resultant side-effects.

Table 19 summarises the primary threats to quality of life attributable to the diagnosis of cancer and its treatment. The extent to which the items listed affect quality of life depends partly on the site of the cancer, the stage of the disease, the type of treatment, and on the likelihood of cure. In this chapter I shall illustrate the way in which a diagnosis of cancer, together with the different treatments, can affect quality of life and describe some of the methods that have been used to measure quality of life in lung cancer, which has a very poor prognosis; breast cancer which has a moderately good prognosis; and testicular cancer which has a relatively good prognosis.

IMPACT OF CANCER DIAGNOSIS ON QUALITY OF LIFE

The mere knowledge of having a life-threatening disease can seriously impair the quality of life. This certainly occurs in individuals who have a good understanding of the implications of the disease, but it is notably worse in those with a poor

TABLE 19

PSYCHOSOCIAL PROBLEMS OF CANCER PATIENTS

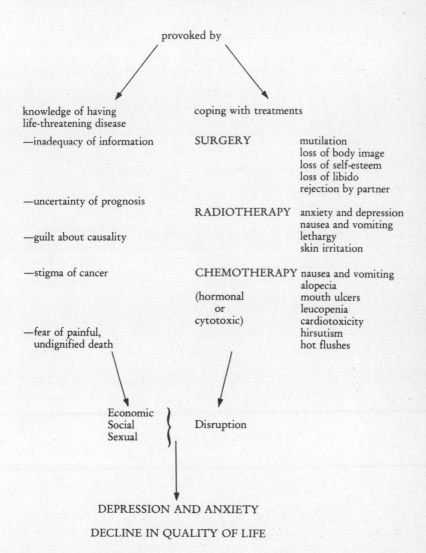

provoked by

knowledge of having
life-threatening disease

—inadequacy of information

—uncertainty of prognosis

—guilt about causality

—stigma of cancer

—fear of painful,
undignified death

coping with treatments

SURGERY   mutilation
                           loss of body image
                           loss of self-esteem
                           loss of libido
                           rejection by partner

RADIOTHERAPY   anxiety and depression
                           nausea and vomiting
                           lethargy
                           skin irritation

CHEMOTHERAPY nausea and vomiting
                           alopecia
(hormonal   mouth ulcers
    or   leucopenia
cytotoxic)   cardiotoxicity
                           hirsutism
                           hot flushes

Economic ⎫
Social   ⎬ Disruption
Sexual   ⎭

DEPRESSION AND ANXIETY

DECLINE IN QUALITY OF LIFE

comprehension of cancer and its treatment. The general public has a large number of serious misconceptions about cancer: most people have curious notions about its causality; many regard it as universally fatal and feel that treatments are basically ineffective; fears that one can catch cancer from a patient with the disease are common, as are worries that death is usually and inevitably preceded by uncontrollable pain. It is extremely important that doctors are made aware of these lay myths and beliefs, as such misinformation can seriously impair a patient's reaction and adjustment to the diagnosis. Such beliefs can also affect the patient's ability or willingness to accept different treatment plans and their tolerance of unpleasant but necessary therapy.

Inadequacy of information
There are innumerable reports in the literature showing that patients with cancer feel dissatisfied with the information given to them by their doctors. For example, in a randomised clinical trial of treatment for early breast cancer, 51 per cent of the patients felt that the information given to them concerning the diagnosis and treatment was inadequate (Fallowfield *et al.*, 1986). In fact, these women had significantly more discussion about treatment options than is usual in a busy out patient clinic, as the study required fully informed consent. When patients were asked what aspects of the information had been inadequate, most acknowledged that hearing the word 'cancer' had so shocked or stunned them that the rest of the conversation was lost. Given the emotionally laden content of the 'bad-news' consultation, this is not an entirely surprising finding. Not only do the patients fail to retain distressing news, but some also repress the information, especially those people who use denial as their primary means of coping.

Quite apart from the legal, moral, or ethical necessity for providing patients with adequate information, there is evidence that well-informed patients are more satisfied with their doctors and more compliant about their treatment. Furthermore, they seem better adjusted to the fact of their cancer. Well-informed patients experience less anxiety and depression when this is measured a year after their diagnosis than those who felt inadequately informed about their disease and treatment (Fallowfield *et al.*, 1986). Despite findings such as these, it is quite common for doctors deliberately to withhold important information on the grounds that they do not wish to upset the patient, or that patients who want to know more will ask. Whilst it is certainly true that brutal, insensitive truth-telling can seriously harm patients, few are helped by some of the euphemisms and pretence employed by certain doctors.

This applies to information about side-effects of treatment as well as the diagnosis. A patient who is not warned about the potential side-effects will mistrust everything else the doctor says. Forewarned means forearmed, so that a patient embarking on chemotherapy, who is warned that she may lose hair and require a wig, will obviously be upset initially, but will be delighted if in fact hair loss is slight. On the other hand, a patient not warned of this possibility, or one who is falsely reassured, will be very distressed and angry if hair loss is in fact significant. She will also lose faith in any future reassurances from that doctor and be constantly worried, sometimes quite needlessly, about things that the doctor may not have told her. Anxious preoccupation with what the doctor really meant can severely impair a patient's ability to enjoy a good quality of life.

Uncertainty of Prognosis
Another frequently heard complaint linked with information giving to patients with cancer is that the doctor was reluctant to provide any prognosis.

A major difficulty for both parties is that there honestly are times when there is little clear information to impart. This is particularly true during the early consultations, prior to confirmation of a cancer diagnosis, whilst awaiting the results of various tests. Anxiety at this time is exacerbated further by those hospital out patient systems where different doctors may see the patient at each visit, all of whom assume that different aspects of the diagnosis, its treatment and probable outcome, have been discussed. It is easy in this situation for some important points to be omitted altogether and for other matters never to be explained properly. Worse still, different doctors may give patients conflicting information about the disease and its likely outcome. As most lay people have a poor understanding about the biology of different cancers and because the outcome of various treatments is sometimes very difficult to predict, patients may misunderstand the doctor's evasiveness about their likely prognosis. Caution can be mistaken for a casual disregard of the patient's plight or indicative of a serious, sinister outcome. Such consultations must be unhurried and handled with deep sensitivity if patients are to feel secure and confident that the doctor has been truthful.

In a study reported by Hogbin and Fallowfield (1989), patients with cancer attending a general surgical out patient department for a consultation about their diagnosis were given audio-tape recordings of this 'bad-news' consultation to take home with them. Despite the emotionally distressing content of the tapes, with cancer being mentioned quite explicitly, patients were overwhelmingly positive about the value of the recordings. Just as some doctors have difficulty breaking bad news to patients, the patients themselves have similar problems conveying this distressing information to their family and friends. As people do not inhabit a social vacuum, the understanding and support of well-informed relatives and friends is extremely important to good long-term adjustment and quality of life. Both patients and their families were deeply appreciative of the efforts to inform them frankly and honestly of the diagnosis and its treatment. It gave them added confidence and trust in the surgeon and his treatment, as can be seen in the following quotation:

> We both appreciated the frank and honest way the doctor spoke to us about cancer. Listening to the tape again gave us great confidence in him. It stopped me feeling so anxious about what was to come.

Stigma of cancer
Along with all the physical and psychological threats to quality of life, the diagnosis of cancer imposes yet another unpleasant burden, that of stigma. Cancer is not a particularly 'hygienic' disease in quite the same way that maybe heart disease or a fractured leg is. It evokes profound sensations of disgust, revulsion and fear in some people, so that the cancer patient becomes a marked person, subjected either implicitly or

explicitly to a number of unfortunate behaviours from others. Even those individuals deemed 'cured' of their cancer still report that the stigma of having experienced this taboo disease remains. Alice Stewart Trillin had adenocarcinoma of the lung when only 36 years old. Four years later, following successful treatment, she described her feelings when she first realised that she had cancer, and the impact that it had on others:

I felt immediately that I had entered a special place, a place I came to call 'The Land of Sick People'. The most disconcerting thing, however, was not that I found that place terrifying and unfamiliar, but that I found it so ordinary, so banal. I didn't feel different, didn't feel that my life had radically changed at the moment the word *cancer* became attached to it. The same rules held. What had changed, however, was other people's perceptions of me. Unconsciously, even with a certain amount of kindness, everyone—with the single rather extraordinary exception of my husband—regarded me as someone who had been altered irrevocably.

I mentioned in Chapter 1 how the perceived withdrawal of others from social contact with cancer sufferers is not merely paranoia on the part of the unfortunate patient, but has an obvious survival advantage in evolutionary terms. In an interesting study on non-cancer sufferers in Germany, Verres (1986) found that although fear of contagion was rarely expressed directly, precise questioning about the degrees of intimacy that people would engage in with a known cancer sufferer showed that over a third would not share utensils used by patients, many would no longer eat anything cooked by someone with cancer and even more avoided any physical contact. However, there are other reasons for this avoidance behaviour, besides fear of contamination: it is deeply depressing to watch someone you know, respect, or love deteriorate physically or mentally, or to witness them suffering from intractable pain. Sometimes our own fear of death is exacerbated by confrontation with anyone who has a life-threatening disease, and thus avoidance of any contact with a potentially dying person helps preserve our own feelings of immortality and invulnerability.

The stigma attached to a diagnosis of cancer is only partially due to the sinister implications that the disease has for the sufferer. Stigma is also a result of the fears evoked by the enigmatic nature of cancer, particularly the uncertainties surrounding its causality and the likely response to therapy. Susan Sontag, in her remarkable book *Illness as Metaphor*, summarised this in the following succinct passage:

> Although the way in which disease mystifies is set against a backdrop of new expectations, the disease itself arouses thoroughly old-fashioned kinds of dread. Any disease that is treated as a mystery and acutely enough feared will be felt morally, if not literally, contagious. Contact with someone afflicted with a disease regarded as a mysterious malevolency inevitably feels like a trespass; worse, like the violation of a taboo.

In 1982, Peters-Golden published results from a questionnaire study of 100 healthy individuals' attitudes to cancer patients and showed that 61 per cent admitted that they would avoid contact with a friend who had cancer. In the same study Peters-Golden found that more than 50 per cent of patients with breast cancer felt that people avoided them and another 70 per cent said that their feelings of social isolation were made more intense because of a lack of understanding by family and friends. As the perceived existence of social support is so crucial to a satisfactory psychological adjustment to cancer (Bloom, 1982), it is important that health educators and others try harder to counter the myths which foster the stigmatising of cancer patients.

Fear of a painful, undignified death

Lay populations in both Europe and the United States consistently overestimate the mortality figures for cancer (Knopf, 1970), so patients for whom cure is a realistic prospect should be reassured to spare them unnecessary fear and anguish. The mental suffering of those patients with a poor prognosis can be ameliorated considerably if they or their relatives are given opportunities to discuss their anxieties about death. When invited to talk about the subject, patients with cancer usually express fears that death will be intolerably painful, that they will lose all control of their bodily functions and that loved ones will abandon them to die alone. Some doctors feel ill-equipped to initiate discussions about topics such as these, and others are less than frank about the putative benefits of further treatments. Professionally trained oncology counsellors can be invaluable at this time.

The degree to which quality of life may be compromised before death is viewed as a preferred state, is undoubtedly a controversial issue, dependent on a number of variables including such things as a patient's religious or philosophical orientation, perceived support from family and friends, as well as clinical judgements. There is often a conflict of interests. The family might put a great deal of pressure on clinicians to preserve life at any cost; patients may feel on balance that they have 'had enough' and wish to be allowed to die in peace; the ambitious, scientific doctor might be reluctant to cease treatment of a patient who is taking part in a controlled clinical trial of a new therapy. Also, many people, both lay and professional, have enormous difficulty in accepting the inevitability of death, so they engage in 'doing something behaviours', that is trying a therapy which in reality has little prospect of either alleviating symptoms or improving survival. Alice Stewart Trillin (1981) has suggested that in this situation 'the patient becomes a kind of talisman for the doctor. Doctors defy death by keeping people alive.'

This displacement activity permits everyone to feel legitimately that they are doing everything they can for the patient. In fact, such behaviour is just side-stepping the primary imperative, which is the necessity for all involved to cease active therapy and to concentrate their efforts on symptomatic relief, especially pain control, together with psychological support for the patient and his or her relatives. Sadly, a neglected but important part of enhancing the quality of life for a person with cancer is to ensure that due concern and attention is paid to the quality of that person's death. This issue will be dealt with more thoroughly in Chapter 8, but it is worth remembering that one of the primary fears attached to the knowledge of having a life-threatening disease is the prospect of suffering a painful, undignified death. The hospice specialists have shown just how dramatically the overall quality of remaining survival can be improved with proper terminal care, with its emphasis on effective pain control and good counselling support for both patients and their families.

IMPACT OF TREATMENTS ON QUALITY OF LIFE

> Diseases desperate grown by desperate appliance are relieved or not at all.   *Hamlet*, Act IV, Sc. iii, l. 9

Cancer is a destructive disease and the treatment methods employed are also destructive, from the cutting and mutilation of surgery to the burning of malignant cells by radiation therapy and the selective poisoning with cytotoxic drugs. In certain cancers, such as the childhood leukaemias and testicular carcinoma, such treatments have improved survival dramatically over the past two decades, but for most of the common solid tumours the picture is still somewhat bleak. Despite the billions of pounds invested in the development and testing of different chemotherapeutic agents, surgical techniques and methods of irradiation, survival statistics have changed very little. Indeed, overtreatment with combination therapy has produced modest extensions in length of survival at great cost to the quality of survival. Undoubtedly there are times when the physical and psychological stress induced by the treatments appears to impair quality of life as much as the disease itself.

The effect of surgery on quality of life

Mutilation
Most people experience anxiety at the prospect of being rendered unconscious and undergoing the 'planned physical assault' of surgery (Gruendemann, 1965). Apart from having to contend with fears about the outcome of the operation, there is the anticipation of post-operative pain and worries about the myriad possible social and economic consequences of a lengthy period of hospitalisation. For the patient with cancer there is the additional burden of possible mutilation and altered bodily functioning. Some malignant tumours require extensive removal of surrounding tissue or the complete extirpation of an organ or limb. Such procedures inevitably cause distress and some patients are never able successfully to

adapt to their altered appearance and/or body function. Unfortunately, those patients who refuse surgery ('I'd rather die than have my breast cut off') may fail to appreciate that untreated cancer producing, for example, an infected, ulcerating growth on the chest wall, can destroy body-image and function in an even more abhorrent manner.

Either way, patients' worries about mutilation must be addressed. It is not sufficient to expect psychological distress to abate with time, in a patient 'grateful' for curative surgery. Patients have a high price to pay for their cure and need understanding, empathetic support and sensible, well-informed advice about prostheses. The partners of patients about to undergo extensive cancer surgery also need good counselling support. It is not logical to invest scarce resources of money and manpower in surgical technology without committing funds to the management of the psychological implications of treatment. A patient 'cured' of his or her cancer, but emotionally crippled because of a distressing appearance or destroyed body function, will not experience a good quality of life unless adequate attention has been given to psychological needs.

Radiotherapy

Unfortunately, high energy irradiation of cancer cells also affects healthy tissue, giving rise to a number of unpleasant and deleterious side-effects. Skin inflammation is common, even with low doses of radiotherapy. At high doses patients can experience permanent changes to skin pigment, skin atrophy and a reduced blood supply, all of which may cause problems with healing if the skin surface is damaged in any way. Nausea, vomiting and diarrhoea are also quite common, especially following irradiation of the abdomen, where the small bowel seems particularly sensitive.

Radiotherapy to the sexual organs can cause many side-effects which severely impair a variety of body functions and quality of life. For example, at high doses irradiation of the ovaries may precipitate an early menopause. Even low doses of radiotherapy to the testes affect the ultra-sensitive sperm-producing cells and cause sterility. Sperm banking may alleviate some of the distress that this can produce. Radiation fibrosis following treatment to the cervix may cause shortening, narrowing and dryness of the vagina, making sexual intercourse painful and unenjoyable.

Irradiation of the head for brain tumours causes hair loss which fails to grow back satisfactorily and usually means that the patient will permanently require a wig. Head and neck cancers nearly always require radiotherapy treatment at some stage and this can cause some painful and unpleasant reactions. For example, secretions in the mouth may diminish and fungal infections are common, making eating a painful and unattractive prospect to someone who may already be experiencing a loss of appetite.

These physical side-effects of radiotherapy are dependent to a certain extent on the site of the cancer, the dosage being administered, and of course the care with which treatment is planned and given. There are many other fairly universal side-effects which can occur, irrespective of cancer site, and these may produce considerable physical and psychological distress. It is not unusual for patients to complain about the unpleasant, persistent, enervating fatigue which accompanies a course of radiotherapy (Fallowfield, 1986, 1988). This extreme tiredness is often worse towards the end of the treatment and can continue for many months, making patients worry that their cancer has not been cured. They may rationalise that if treatment has been successful, then why are they feeling so dreadful? One contributory factor to the overwhelming fatigue is the fact that radiotherapy is only provided in specialist centres, so some patients are required to travel long distances daily for several weeks. Other patients have to be admitted to hospital for treatment, either because they live too far away or because they are receiving radiation from an implant rather than by external beam. Being away from home can in itself create considerable anxiety at a time when patients are most in need of social support.

Another disagreeable feature of treatment is that of lengthy waiting periods, often in somewhat gloomy, uninviting and inadequately furbished departments. Talking to other patients awaiting treatment, some of whom may be seriously ill, with recurrent disease or having palliative treatment for advanced cancer, can be profoundly depressing and some patients become extremely fearful that they will share a similarly unpleasant fate. Patients are inclined to be unduly pessimistic about radiotherapy anyway. One study by Peck and Boland (1977) showed that few of the 50 patients whom they interviewed realised that radiotherapy is often curative.

One often underestimated anxiety is the patients' fear that the treatment being given to cure their cancer, paradoxically, is linked with causing cancer also. The warning notices displayed everywhere in radiotherapy departments, together with the fact that everyone involved with delivering therapy retreats behind thick concrete walls and lead shields, does little to alleviate worries that the procedure is dangerous. There is some evidence that patients treated with the fast, linear accelerator machines rather than the slow, older, noisy betatron apparatus, seem to experience less psychological distress during therapy (Forester *et al.*, 1978).

The complex interactions between the psychological and physical aspects associated with radiotherapy are both interesting and important to understand if patients are to be helped through the ordeal. The mere knowledge that one is having radiotherapy can provoke side-effects. Parsons *et al.* (1961) found that 75 per cent of patients receiving 'sham' radiotherapy nonetheless experienced nausea and fatigue.

Despite the large number of unwanted side-effects mentioned in this section, all of which impact on quality of life, good quality radiotherapy treatment can often cure those cancers that are impossible to remove surgically. It can sometimes be offered to patients as an adequate alternative to surgery, which will not compromise survival and avoids mutilation. Radiotherapy can also palliate advanced cancer, bringing welcome pain relief to patients suffering the intense pain caused by bony secondaries, and can shrink those tumours which may be preventing patients swallowing or breathing properly. Quality of life during the unpleasant period of radiotherapy treatment could probably be enhanced by such things as an efficient appointments system and upgrading of the waiting areas in radiotherapy departments. Good information from well-trained staff about the possible side-effects and means of coping with them is imperative, and provision of an oncology counselling service for patients and their families would permit the amelioration of fears and anxieties about therapy. These should also be seen as an important, necessary adjunct to treatment if the quality of life and sense of well-being is to be preserved in patients with cancer.

Chemotherapy

Of all the treatments given to treat cancer, systemic therapy with cytotoxic agents probably has the worst reputation. Given the vast litany of severe side-effects which can occur, this reputation is richly deserved. Unfortunately these side-effects are inevitable; chemotherapeutic agents not only kill the rapidly multiplying cancer cells, but also those other, normal cells of the body characterised by rapid cell division. Cells within the hair follicles, bone marrow and lining of the gastrointestinal tract are particularly vulnerable, hence the well-known side-effects of alopecia, bleeding, anaemia, lowered resistance to infection, vomiting and diarrhoea. Less well-known to the patients, but a considerable worry to the clinician, are cardiotoxicity and neurotoxicity—problems affecting the heart, lungs and nervous system. There are numerous reports in the literature showing, not surprisingly, that the greater the toxicity, the higher the emotional distress and diminution of quality of life. Some cytotoxic drugs affect the brain biochemistry directly, which results in mood disturbances and other cognitive impairments (Silberfarb *et al.*, 1980).

Nausea and vomiting are the commonest of the unpleasant side-effects associated with chemotherapy. Patients, who may cope well with the embarrassment of alopecia and the miseries of bowel upset or mouth soreness, find nausea and vomiting such an intolerable burden that they may refuse to complete treatment. One survey of specialist cancer centres in the United States of America revealed that in 80 per cent of the hospitals, as many as ten per cent of their patients refused further treatment because of the distress it caused (Penta *et al.*, 1981).

As some of the cytotoxics produce such a powerful emetic effect, the behaviour can quickly become a classically conditioned response. Any of the stimuli associated with chemotherapy, for example the nurses, the hospital, needles, the word 'chemotherapy', or even the mere thought of going for treatment, may elicit nausea and vomiting. This distressing experience can persist long after treatment ceases. One breast cancer patient told me that she still continued to vomit whenever she passed the hospital where she had received her chemotherapy some two years previously.

The number of patients for whom chemotherapy produces anticipatory nausea and/or vomiting varies depending on the type of cytotoxic agent or combination of agents being given. Most well-controlled studies show that it is a significant problem, impairing the quality of life for between 24 and 38 per cent of all patients (Mohrer *et al.*, 1984). In another interesting study, Coates and his colleagues (1983) gave patients undergoing different cytotoxic therapy 73 cards on which were written various side-effects, symptoms and problems. There were 45 physical problem cards and 28 non-physical, psychosocial problem cards, which patients were instructed to rank in order of severity. All groups gave nausea and vomiting top ranking as the worst side-effect, but those patients receiving cisplatin gave 'thought of coming for treatment' second rating. These patients were given the drug lorazepam for both its anxiolytic and amnesic effects and were thus helped through their treatment more successfully. Fortunately, psychologists have also developed some behavioural inventions which can help ameliorate the amount of nausea and vomiting endured in anticipation of and during treatment (Morrow and Morrow, 1982).

Curative Chemotherapy
Developing ways to help patients cope with some of the most distressing side-effects of chemotherapy is vital, as certain cancers, in particular testicular cancer, Hodgkin's disease and many childhood leukaemias, can be completely cured with aggressive treatment. Unfortunately, the price patients have to pay for cure is toleration of the side-effects from extremely high doses of cytotoxic drugs, together with other psychosocial problems. The stress involved may even cause marital breakups. Fobair *et al.* (1986) reported high rates of divorce amongst Hodgkin's disease patients who underwent aggressive chemotherapy and concluded that '. . . during this time couples found it almost impossible to face their anger, especially the

understandable but irrational anger felt by the healthy spouse toward the ill one for becoming sick and thereby disrupting both lives. Most spouses felt comfortable expressing such resentments only after the treatment was completed, when the patient seemed strong enough to take it.'

Adjuvant Chemotherapy

Chemotherapy is sometimes given as an adjuvant to patients who have already undergone surgical removal of a tumour. Side-effects in this situation are poorly tolerated as the patient is usually still feeling physically and emotionally burdened by the operation, and the need for further treatment such as radiotherapy or chemotherpy serves to reinforce the idea that the cancer has not been completely removed. Comments by the doctor that chemotherapy is being given 'to clear up any remaining cancer cells floating around' produce considerable anxiety. Maguire et al. (1980) studied the psychological effect of giving cyclophosphamide, methotrexate and 5-fluorouracil (CMF) after treatment for breast cancer by mastectomy. Anxiety and/or depression was evident in many of the women so treated, especially in those who also experienced the most physical side-effects. In all, 20 out of 26 women who received chemotherapy developed psychiatric morbidity and this was significantly higher than the psychological distress of the comparison group who underwent mastectomy without adjuvant chemotherapy.

Palliative Chemotherapy

The use of unpleasant toxic chemotherapy in patients for whom palliation, not cure, is the only goal, arouses deep and bitter controversy. This is the area where good quality of life assessment has an invaluable role to play in guiding treatment decisions and evaluating the therapeutic outcome of different drug regimens. The sole purpose of giving any treatment to patients with advanced metastatic disease is, after all, to palliate symptoms and thus improve the quality of life left. Too often this goal is lost sight of by enthusiasts who see increased survival time as the primary imperative. In some forms of metastatic lung cancer, for example, it is difficult to envisage how any net benefit can accrue to a patient who may

gain a modest extension of survival with aggressive chemotherapy, if those few precious extra months are spent
experiencing debilitating nausea and vomiting, hair loss,
mouth soreness and hospitalisation for treatments (Aisner *et
al.*, 1981). Indeed, the use of cytotoxics in the treatment of
most of the common solid tumours seems difficult to defend
when the impact that side-effects exerted upon quality of life
are considered.

Doctors have a duty to be much more honest with
themselves and their patients about the actual therapeutic
benefits of chemotherapy. Some patients will still be altruistic
enough to embark on experimental therapy when in the
terminal stages of disease. They gain some satisfaction from
the knowledge that through their own suffering others may be
helped. However, patients for whom palliation is the only
realistic aim need a frank but sensitive discussion about the
limitations of chemotherapy, together with thorough, positive
counselling and advice about the symptomatic relief and
supportive treatments which can be offered instead. This is
also a time when relatives need to be convinced that trips
around the world with the hapless patient, in search of a
wonder drug, are not in the patient's best interests.

Hormonal Chemotherapy
Because of its relative lack of toxicity, hormonal chemotherapy
has a much gentler image than cytotoxic therapy. One
advantage of its usage is that it may improve mood state in
certain patients; for example Twycross and Guppy (1985)
found that prednisolone enhanced the sense of well-being and
raised the spirits of patients with terminal breast and lung
cancer. The development of drugs such as tamoxifen has been a
major breakthrough. Tamoxifen is extremely effective in
improving both the length of survival and quality of life of
patients with breast cancer, without producing the intolerable
side-effects found following cytotoxic chemotherapy or some
other hormonal steroids. The hormonal preparations used
prior to the advent of tamoxifen could produce weight-again,
steroidal 'moon-face', changes in the distribution of body fat
and hair, producing hirsutism, virilism or feminisation, all of
which could be profoundly distressing for sick people who

might have already had to cope with an altered body-image following mutilating surgery. Some hormonal therapy for prostatic cancer causes impotence, and it can affect libido when given to patients with prostatic, uterine or breast cancer.

*   *   *

Patients with cancer have to come to terms with the knowledge that they have a life-threatening disease and must develop strategies to cope with the treatments. All these things can disrupt economic, social and sexual functioning and frequently cause anxiety and depression, thus diminishing quality of life.

Even if we do reduce the toxicity of treatments and can increase disease-free survival, I would like to suggest that the psychological impact of having had a diagnosis of cancer and having suffered during therapy is likely to manifest itself as a major long-term complication of cancer treatment. Fobair *et al.* (1986), for example, interviewed 403 patients who were approximately one year post-treatment for Hodgkin's disease. Thirty-seven per cent of their sample were still suffering from persistent energy loss (the remainder had required between 12 and 16 months for energy to return to normal). Those suffering a self-reported energy loss were also more likely to be depressed. Divorce rates were high (32 per cent) and 20 per cent of the patients still had a loss of sexual interest. Forty-two per cent had employment difficulties and this again seemed to correlate with depression and energy loss. Clearly, it is not sufficient to assume that curing cancer relieves patients of the major psychosocial problems which affect quality of life. Adequate assessment of the outcome of treatment is necessary, whether cure or palliation is the goal. This also allows psychologists and counsellors to develop appropriate inter-ventions to assist patients and their families during and following therapy.

So what are the key areas of quality of life in cancer in general that require monitoring? What are the problems specific to certain types of malignancy and their treatment? And what are the most useful measures of quality of life in cancer?

Depression and Anxiety

Depression and anxiety are extremely common emotional disturbances found in patients with cancers. Studies of adult cancer patients demonstrate that between 24 and 56 per cent (Derogatis *et al.*, 1983, Bukberg *et al.*, 1984) experience clinically significant signs of depression, and furthermore that these problems may be unremitting without treatment. The prevalence estimates amongst patients vary depending on the site of the cancer, the diagnostic criteria and assessment measures employed. However, the primary symptom demanded for a diagnosis of depression is unremitting, persistent lowering of mood and sadness of at least four weeks' duration. This, together with a constellation of other symptoms such as guilt, lowering of self-esteem, suicidal ideation, hopelessness about the future, impaired memory and concentration, irritability, appetite changes, loss of libido, insomnia, fatigue and psychomotor retardation or agitation, forms the diagnostic criterion for depression in the Diagnostic and Statistical Manual (DSM III) of the American Psychiatric Association (APA 1980). Using the same diagnostic manual, anxiety state requires the presence of one primary mood disorder, that is persistent feelings of tension and apprehension or an inability to relax of at least four weeks' duration, together with four other symptoms such as sleep disturbance, impaired concentration, fatigability, somatic symptoms (headaches, sweating, palpitations, tremor), panic attacks or irritability. One difficulty when assessing patients who are physically ill is that many of the somatic symptoms used for a diagnosis of depression and/or anxiety may be part of the cancer itself or due to the treatment. Some clinicians have suggested, therefore, that more emphasis should be placed on the non-somatic components of mood disorders when assessing patients already in a physically compromised state due to cancer (Plum and Holland, 1981).

Semi-structured psychiatric interviews, such as the Hamilton Rating Scale for Depression (1967) or the shortened version of the Present State Examination (PSE) of Wing *et al.* (1974), have been used successfully to rate depression and anxiety in cancer patients. The most frequently used Hamilton Scale includes 17 items assessing cognitive, behavioural and physiological signs and symptoms of depression, although there is another 20-item version tapping feelings of hopelessness, helplessness and worthlessness, which may be relevant for use with cancer patients. Unfortunately, such semi-structured assessments are time-consuming and demand a well-trained interviewer. It is more appropriate in a busy oncology clinic, therefore, to use self-assessment questionnaires: good examples are the General Health Questionnaire (see Chapter 2), the Wakefield or Beck Depression Inventories and the Spielberger State Trait Anxiety Scale (1968). However, all these tests were designed for use with non-medically sick individuals, so threshold scores may require some adjustment. Probably a better way to screen cancer patients for signs of a mood disorder that should be investigated further is with the Hospital Anxiety and Depression Scale (HAD) developed by Zigmond and Snaith (1983), which I have already described in Chapter 2. Its advantage over the other self-assessment questionnaires is that all the items contained within the scale deal with emotional, not physical symptoms.

One final point worth mentioning is that the mood disorder found amongst cancer patients is not always a reactive depression due to the stress associated with the illness or other unpleasant life events in the social milieu. Depression can be due to organic brain syndromes produced by such things as cerebral metastases or metabolic upset, caused by liver failure or hypercalcaemia, and drugs, especially steroids and cytotoxics.

There are still too many doctors who feel that depression and anxiety are to be expected in association with cancer and that these 'normal' reactions do not therefore merit treatment. This is as nonsensical as saying that as pain is a 'normal' reaction to surgery it does not require analgesia. The quality of life of many emotionally distressed patients can be greatly improved if they are referred on for help from a properly trained oncology counsellor or to an interested psychiatrist who may embark on a course of psychotherapy, supplemented with anti-depressant and/or anxiolytic drugs. Prophylactic counselling may help prevent the obsessional anxiety shown by some patients who exhibit hypervigilant monitoring of their bodies for signs and symptoms of the dreaded recurrence.

QUALITY OF LIFE IN SPECIFIC MALIGNANCIES

Cancer with a poor prognosis

More than 40,000 men and women in the United Kingdom die each year of lung cancer. Table 18 (p. 76) showed that the five-year survival rate is very poor. Thus, many patients have to cope with the fact that their cancer is likely to prove fatal. One means of preserving hope and coping with such unpalatable facts is the strategy of denial. In an interesting study of 183 patients with inoperable lung cancer, Jones (1981) gave patients the option of full information concerning their prognosis. Of the 90 patients who asked, ten subsequently 'denied' the knowledge and reality of their disease. A further 93 patients never asked, but it was clear at a later interview that at least half of them knew the probable outcome. In another study of 50 inoperable lung cancer patients, Hughes (1985) reported that 19 of the sample claimed that they anticipated a complete recovery from their disease and none of these patients showed any signs of depression. A major depressive illness was apparent in six of the 20 patients who expressed awareness of a fatal outcome.

Some of the depression found amongst lung cancer patients is almost certainly due to the unpleasantly toxic chemotherapy given and the effects that some drugs have on central neurotransmitters. Silberfarb et al. (1983) gave the Profile of Mood States (POMS) shown in Chapter 2 to patients receiving different cytotoxic chemotherapy regimens for small cell lung cancer. They reported no difference in survival between groups, but found that those patients who received combination chemotherapy containing Vincristine suffered significantly more depression and fatigue.

In an impressive multicentre, collaborative randomised clinical trial of different treatment regimens in small cell lung carcinoma involving 30 hospitals throughout Europe, the European Organisation for Research and Treatment of Cancer (EORTC) developed a multidimensional self-assessment questionnaire to assess quality of life (Aaronson, 1987). The EORTC questionnaire assesses functioning in physical, psychological and social domains forming a 'core' questionnaire. Its novelty over other measures is that it also has a lung cancer specific module which addresses issues particularly relevant to patients who may have problems with breathing, the side-effects of chemotherapy and pain control (see Table 20). Hopefully, the meticulous care with which the authors are evaluating and refining their instrument (Aaronson et al., 1988) will not only provide important information regarding the quality of life with different treatment regimens in non-resectable lung cancer, but will also prove to be a major breakthrough in the standardisation of assessment methods in cancer clinical trials. The complete results of this lung cancer trial have not yet been published, but some early data have shown, for example, significant psychological distress: 'tension' was reported by 45 per cent of the sample, and 'worrying' by 44 per cent; 'depression' was a problem for 34 per cent and irritability for 21 per cent of the patients (Aaronson et al., 1987).

Other studies have suggested that patients with lung cancer are more likely to have a poorer quality of life than other cancer patients in view of the emotional trauma of having a cancer with a grave prognosis, the self-remorse and guilt about having 'caused' the cancer by smoking, the pain and anorexia from metastatic spread of the disease and the side-effects of chemotherapy. Weisman and Worden (1977), for example, found that people with a past history of psychological problems, patients at an advanced stage of disease at diagnosis and people with a diagnosis of lung cancer were most likely to have serious emotional difficulties and coping problems. Houts et al. (1986) in the United States interviewed 629 people with cancer to determine their unmet psychological, social and economic needs. People with lung cancer reported significantly more unmet needs in every category investigated, suggesting that they experienced a poorer quality of life than did patients with other forms of cancer.

Cancer with a moderately good prognosis
Breast cancer is the biggest killer of western women. There are 24,500 new cases diagnosed each year in the United Kingdom and more than 15,000 women die from it. Despite these gloomy statistics, breast cancer, especially early stage disease, does have a moderately good prognosis. Table 18 (p. 76) shows

TABLE 20
THE EORTC LUNG CANCER MODULE

Patients sometimes report that they have the following symptoms. Please indicate the extent to which you have experienced these symptoms during the past week.

During the past week:	Not at all	A little	Quite a bit	Very much
37 How much did you cough?	1	2	3	4
38 Did you cough blood?	1	2	3	4
39 Were you short of breath when you rested?	1	2	3	4
40 Were you short of breath when you walked?	1	2	3	4
41 Were you short of breath when you climbed stairs?	1	2	3	4
42 Have you had a sore mouth or tongue?	1	2	3	4
43 Have you had trouble swallowing?	1	2	3	4
44 Have you had tingling hands or feet?	1	2	3	4
45 Have you been bothered by hair loss?	1	2	3	4
46 Have you had pain in the chest?	1	2	3	4
47 Have you had pain in your arm or shoulder?	1	2	3	4
48 Have you had pain in other parts of your body?	1	2	3	4
If yes, where?				

_____

	Not at all	A little	Quite a bit	Very much
49 Did you take any medicine for pain?				
1 No				
2 Yes—how much did it help?	1	2	3	4

Please check to make sure that you have answered all of the questions.

that the five-year relative survival rate is 62 per cent. However, it is very important to examine the quality of that survival. Because of the high incidence of breast cancer, and the repugnance with which mastectomy is held, there have been numerous studies measuring aspects of the quality of life.

Consistent reports have appeared in the medical literature and lurid accounts in the lay press, highlighting the psychological havoc wreaked by surgical treatment of breast cancer involving amputation of the breast and surrounding tissues—mastectomy. Most of these reports assumed that the high incidence of depression, anxiety and sexual dysfunction was due to the severe assault on body image. Sutherland (1967), for example, wrote that 'Mastectomy is an intolerable insult to women whose self-esteem and expectation of esteem from others is predicated to a large extent on their beauty and shapeliness'. This is undoubtedly true, given the powerfully symbolic nature of the breast in our culture, linked as it is to feelings of femininity, sexuality and motherhood. However, the emphasis given to breast loss rather than the fact of having cancer has probably been over-stated. Peters-Golden (1982) examined the perceptions held by patients and non-patients about breast cancer. It was considered 'the worst thing that can happen to a woman' by 59 per cent of the men interviewed, whilst only six per cent of patients thought this to be true.

Two of the earliest methodologically sound studies were conducted in the United Kingdom by Morris *et al.* (1977) and Maguire *et al.* (1978). Using either the Wakefield Psychiatric Rating Scale or a modified version of the Present State Examination (PSE), both studies established that women who had been treated for breast cancer by mastectomy had significantly higher rates of anxiety and/or depression than control groups a year or more post-operation. This psychiatric morbidity post-mastectomy is made worse if adjuvant chemotherapy is given. Palmer *et al.* (1980) used a self-rating questionnaire to compare an aggressive cytotoxic regimen with low toxicity single-agent chemotherapy. The greater the objective toxicity of the chemotherapy, the more adverse were the effects on quality of life.

In a rather different study of women receiving treatments for advanced breast cancer, quality of life was monitored using the LASA (see Chapter 2), Priestman and Baum (1978) found that although patients receiving cytotoxic chemotherapy experienced more treatment-related side-effects than those receiving hormonal therapy, overall well-being was significantly better in the cytotoxic therapy group. This paradoxical result was explained by the fact that those women who had the cytotoxic therapy experienced significantly better objective response rates. The side-effects of treatment were therefore offset by the symptomatic relief experienced with tumour shrinkage.

The intuitive assumptions made by many people that techniques to treat breast cancer, which do not demand extensive mutilating surgery, would result in a better quality of life without compromising survival, have not been realised. There are to date no firm data showing an advantage with breast conservation and radiotherapy. There is evidence that mastectomy causes extreme distress and considerable psychiatric morbidity in those women for whom body image is their primary focus of concern, but the majority of women are more concerned about getting rid of their cancer.

In a randomised controlled clinical trial of treatment for early breast cancer, I interviewed 101 women using the PSE. The patients also filled in two self-assessment questionnaires, the HAD and the RSCL described in Chapter 2. The incidence of depressive illness and/or anxiety among women who underwent mastectomy was high (33 per cent) and comparable to that found in other studies. The surprise and disappointment to many was that slightly more of the women who underwent a lumpectomy followed by radiotherapy (38 per cent) experienced anxiety and/or depression (Fallowfield et al., 1986). Although the mastectomy-treated women expressed more overt concern about appearance and the effect that their surgery might be having on sexual relationships, there was in fact no difference in sexual interest between the two groups. The RSCL showed that 38 per cent of women, irrespective of treatment, reported somewhat or very much of a lack of sexual interest. Indeed, on several items of the RSCL, the lumpectomy patients were significantly more anxious than the mastectomy patients (Fallowfield et al., 1987). This anxiety seemed to stem from a feeling of uncertainty about the prognosis and the constant awareness of a possible recurrence. Some women admitted to compulsive checking of their breasts for other lumps. The following extract from a taped interview demonstrates these problems:

'Do you know, if I get a pain in my stomach now it's got to be cancer; if I've got a pain in my back I'm going to get lung cancer; get a bad head, I'm getting a tumour on the brain. I just can't get it out of my head.

'I just cannot keep my hand off (my breast). It's something that I've never, ever done. I spend hours just lying there feeling, and when I touch I feel as if I've got lumps all over.' (Quoted from Fallowfield *et al.*, 1986.)

Table 21 shows that there are to date ten published studies comparing quality of life in patients treated for breast cancer by mastectomy or breast-conserving procedures. Despite the large number of assessment methods employed, one clear finding emerges, which is that there is no improvement in quality of life following lumpectomy, although a small advantage in terms of body image is seen in five of the studies. The impact that a diagnosis of cancer has on quality of life is not necessarily ameliorated by sparing the women the trauma of breast loss. This finding is analogous to those found in quality of life studies in patients with soft tissue and bone carcinoma. Research has shown that survival is similar, irrespective of treatment offered, which can be either limb amputation or limb salvage with chemotherapy and radio-therapy. Limb preservation techniques have grown in popularity due to the assumption that they would convey a superior quality of life in terms of psychological and social benefits to patients. At least two studies using assessments, including the PAIS, SIP, POMS, ADL (all described in Chapter 2) and many other tests, reported the seemingly counterintuitive finding that there was no difference between groups. Limb salvage is complex; it requires longer hospitalisation than amputation; there is a high risk of neurovascular damage and necrosis and the preserved limb often functions rather poorly. Just as I found with the women who had had breast-conserving procedures, many of the limb salvage patients complained that they felt constantly anxious that the cancer would return and were poorly adjusted to their illness (Sugarbaker *et al.*, 1982, Weddington *et al.*, 1985).

TABLE 21

Studies comparing psychological outcome of mastectomy and breast conversion

Authors	Number of Patients	Assessments Used	Primary Findings
Sanger & Reznikoff	40 mastectomy (20) breast conservation (20)	Rorschach ink-blots Locke & Wallace Marital Adjustment (MAT) Secord Homonyms test & Body Cathexis Scale MMPI Crowne-Marlow Social Desirability	No significant differences between groups on 'body anxiety', psychological adjustment or marital satisfaction. Greater overall 'body satisfaction' in conservatively treated group
Schain et al (1983)	38 mastectomy (20) excisional biopsy (18)	Non-standard self-report questionnaire	No significant psychosocial differences, but less negative body image in breast conservation group
Ashcroft et al (1985)	40 mastectomy lumpectomy (numbers unknown)	Leeds Depression Scale Spielberger Trait Anxiety Inventory (STAI) Locke & Wallace MATS Holmes & Rahe Life Events Schedule	Little difference between groups on psychosocial measures but better body satisfaction in breast conservation group

TABLE 21 (continued)

Authors	Number of Patients	Assessments Used	Primary Findings
Bartelink et al (1985)	172 radical mastectomy (58) breast conservation (114)	Non-standard 9-item self-report questionnaire	Less negative body image and fear of recurrence in breast conservation group
de Haes et al (1986)	41 mastectomy (18) tumorectomy (21)	Cancer Patients' Symptom Checklist Non-standard tests of:- body image, marital satisfaction, fear of recurrence and death	Less negative body image in tumorectomy group. No differences in sexual or psychological functioning or in fear of recurrence or death
Fallowfield et al (1986)	101 mastectomy (53) lumpectomy (48)	Present State Examination (PSE) Rotterdam Symptom Checklist (RSCL) Hospital Anxiety & Depression Scale (HAD)	No difference in psychiatric morbidity betwen groups, but more overt concern with fear of cancer recurrence amongst lumpectomy patients
Lasry et al (1987)	123 mastectomy (43) lumpectomy plus radiation (36) lumpectomy (44)	CES-Depression Scale Non-standard body image index	Depression highest in lumpectomy patients who also had radiotherapy. Better body image in lumpectomy group. Fear of recurrence greatest amongst patients receiving chemotherapy.

TABLE 21 (continued)

Authors	Number of Patients	Assessments Used	Primary Findings
Wolberg et al (1987)	206 mastectomy (96) (no choice) mastectomy (56) (choice) breast conservation (54) (choice)	Profile of Mood States (POMS) Health Locus of Control (HLOC) Locke-Wallace (MAT) Psychosocial Adjustment to Illness Scale (PAIS) Derogatis Sexual Functioning Inventory (DSFI) and other tests	Psychosocial data (reported from maximum of only 39 patients in original sample) showed advantages to women who elected to have breast conservation in terms of anxiety and depression
Morris et al (1988)	30 mastectomy (10) (no choice) mastectomy 7 (choice) wide excision (13)	Hospital Anxiety and Depression Scale (HAD) Rotterdam Symptom Checklist (RSCL)	No difference in psychiatric morbidity between lumpectomy and mastectomy. Patients not offered choice of treatment more depressed and anxious.
Kenny et al (1988)	52 mastectomy (27) segmentectomy (25)	Non-standard questionnaire Brief Symptom Inventory (BSI) (developed by authors)	No significant differences between mastectomy and segmentectomy patients in 'psychologic symptomatology'. Body image benefit to segmentectomy patients.

Cancer with a good prognosis

Testicular cancer affects relatively few people in the United Kingdom each year (approximately 1,000), but it is the most common malignancy found in men between the ages of 15 and 35 years. Although the latest available figures reveal that 146 young men died of the disease in 1986 (CRC, 1988), the relative five-year survival rate is extremely favourable. Provided that the tumours are discovered at an early stage, without evidence of advanced metastatic spread, at least 90 per cent of all new cases can realistically expect to be cured. (In many forms of testicular cancer this cure rate approaches 100 per cent.) These figures are impressive when one considers the bleak outlook 25 years ago, when the majority of men with the disease were dead within five years. These improvements are due to the significant advances in the clinical management of testicular cancer. Modern computer-aided diagnostic procedures (tomography), together with sophisticated blood tests, permit very accurate staging of the disease, which can then help to determine the most appropriate management. Although radiotherapy still has a role to play in the treatment of testicular cancer, together with surgery, the major breakthrough has come about with the advent of extremely effective cytotoxic chemotherapeutic agents. Unfortunately, patients must suffer a considerable number of side-effects from the aggressive chemotherapy necessary to effect a cure, but most patients seem prepared to tolerate these unpleasant high dose regimens if cure is a realistic goal.

Effective treatment for testicular cancer is available, but those young men unfortunate enough to require such therapy have to contend with several threats to quality of life. Many of the items shown in Table 19 (p. 77) are applicable: the knowledge of having cancer, fear and embarrassment, especially as the cancer involves such an important, intimate site; problems with body image following orchiectomy (surgical removal of the testicle); worries about sexual potency and the numerous side-effects that accompany radiotherapy and chemotherapy.

Psychiatric Morbidity

I have discussed the fact that cancer, irrespective of site, carries with it high levels of psychiatric morbidity. Most studies using a variety of measures, from self-support questionnaires to clinical interviews, show that between 20 and 35 per cent of all cancer patients experience anxiety and/or depression. One might expect that in those cancers with an excellent prognosis, such as testicular cancer, these rates would be much lower. Results from research projects do not support this hypothesis. Moynihan (1987), using the PSE, reported that 23 per cent of patients demonstrated psychiatric morbidity. In the younger patients, i.e. those under 20 years, this figure was 58 per cent. Psychiatric morbidity was not related to the extent of the disease, but patients receiving the most toxic chemotherapy had the highest levels of psychological distress.

Sexual Difficulties
There are some conflicting results from studies addressing the psychosexual sequelae of treatment for testicular cancer. This is probably due to different assessment measures being employed, together with a wide range of time between treatment and evaluation. Schrover and Von Eschenbach (1985), for example, reported a high incidence of sexual and relationship difficulties amongst testicular cancer patients, and Rieker *et al.* (1985), in an extensive study of 74 patients, found that almost 50 per cent of the men were experiencing sexual difficulties, especially with ejaculation. In the latter study, the sexual impairment was correlated with marital disharmony and psychological distress as measured by the POMS. Moynihan (1987) reported that in her sample of 122 men, 29 per cent 'had noticed a deterioration in sexual function since diagnosis, although no patient classified this as a "serious" problem.' She also found no correlation between sexual difficulty and psychiatric morbidity. One explanation for the differences in perception of sexual problems between the two studies mentioned earlier and those of Moynihan could be linked with the fact that in the United States many patients with testicular cancer undergo more radical surgery, which can affect ejaculation. Routine dissection of the retroperineal lymph nodes is not common practice in the United Kingdom.

Fertility

Although a few men may have problems achieving an erection, the majority have no difficulty and most can ejaculate. However, many men are extremely worried about their ability to father children following treatment. Psychiatric morbidity appears higher in men who are uncertain about their fertility, irrespective of whether or not they have banked sperm prior to treatment. Chemotherapy does cause sterility, but this usually reverts to normal within a year or two. Fears that there might be a higher incidence of congenital abnormalities in the children of men who have undergone aggressive therapy have not been substantiated. Both Rieker *et al.* (1985) and Moynihan (1987) have shown that worries about fertility contribute to psychological distress in men with testicular cancer, even if sexual performance is unimpaired.

Body Image

Patients with cancer at other sites who require mutilating surgery often have problems with altered body image. In general, body image concerns do not appear to be amongst the primary worries of men with cancer of the testes. In Moynihan's study few men accepted the offer of a prosthesis. Most claimed that the loss of a testicle had not undermined their manhood and that they felt that their wives and girlfriends showed understanding of the situation. Hair loss during chemotherapy can be devastating for certain patients; however, in the past decade some young men have been able to respond less negatively towards alopecia as shaven heads have been fashionable.

*   *   *

The fact that psychological distress, which profoundly affects quality of life, is still so apparent in cancer patients who have an extremely good prospect of complete cure may seem counterintuitive but demonstrates the need for good counselling support, irrespective of cancer site.

THE APPEAL OF UNORTHODOX QUACK CURES IN CANCER

Unscrupulous practitioners have not been slow in seizing the opportunity to capitalise on our inability to cure all cancers, hence the profusion of quack cures and remedies. The American Cancer Society (1982) categorised more than 70 different unproven methods which include diets, drugs and pseudo-psychological approaches, many complete with their own diagnostic paraphernalia and testing devices. These alternative treatments range from the merely benign or faintly ridiculous, through to the positively harmful, none of which either improve or extend the quality of cancer patients' lives.

All of these quack cures and remedies share two defining characteristics, namely that they are invariably expensive and also ineffective. The pedlars of unproven methods, be they charlatans or merely misguided, are taking advantage of that vital human need to maintain hope in the face of tragedy. Quack cures are rarely evident for treatable disease. The unscrupulous, alternative practitioners are successful in promotion of the myth that they have some miraculous solutions that have been either missed or deliberately ignored by orthodox medicine. Few patients find it easy to accept that they have a terminal disease and relatives likewise wish to believe in miracles. Thus the opportunists actively collude with these desperate and vulnerable sick people in perpetrating a forlorn hope that cure is still possible.

The extent to which patients with cancer are prepared to accept unproven methods is a reflection of dissatisfaction with predominantly two areas of orthodox cancer care—1) the loss of control; and 2) poor communication and support.

1   Loss of Control

Most cancer therapies involve high technology, not only for the delivery of treatments such as surgery, radiotherapy and chemotherapy, but also for diagnosis such as bone scans. Patients are often frightened by these and furthermore feel that things are completely beyond their control. Not only do they feel that the cancer itself has taken control of their bodies, but that the doctors have done so as well. Part of the attraction of alternative therapies is the fact that they appear gentler, less toxic and that they give back to the patients a sense of mastery and self respect—all of which contribute to an enhancement of quality of life. The stranger the dietary regimen, involving not only the patient, but his or her family as well in complex preparations, the more this sense of maintaining control is fostered. A report by Cassileth (1984) stated that 37 per cent of all cancer patients studied were receiving some form of unorthodox dietary regime as well as orthodox therapy (Cassileth, 1984).

2   Poor Communication and Support

Patients and their families often fall prey to alternative practitioners if disillusioned by the inability of more orthodox medical practitioners to communicate effectively. The frequently reported failure of the latter to provide the necessary support required to cope with having a fatal illness, which includes allowing patients either to opt out of aggressive therapy or to volunteer for participation in clinical trials, also makes patients easy game for the unscrupulous.

SUMMARY

The plethora of physical and psychosocial problems confronting patients with cancer, which have such a deleterious impact on quality of life, cannot be adequately summarised in just one chapter. I hope that I have managed to convey the extent of the problem and the need for quality of life measures to play a central role in determining the response to treatment. Interested readers may find helpful a review by Clark and Fallowfield (1986) containing further tests for measuring quality of life in malignant disease. Research continues to validate and standardise self-assessment schedules to assess quality of life in cancer. This is extremely important, as funds for the routine screening and monitoring of patients by trained oncology counsellors are unlikely to be available in the current economic climate.

Some clinicians have little genuine respect for the efforts of those concerned with psychosocial care and pay only lip-service to the concept of quality of life. They have a responsibility to be much more honest with themselves and their patients about the true therapeutic benefits of certain treatments. When palliation is the only realistic aim, it seems quite unethical to put patients through the traumas of cytotoxic therapy which will probably only impair the quality of remaining life, with little real hope of extending survival. Cancer is a very cruel disease and treatments impose a great physical and emotional burden on patients. Likewise, the stresses of dealing with cancer patients can provoke feelings of disillusionment, inadequacy and sorrow on the part of the carers. The quality of life of everyone working in the demanding field of cancer can suffer if adequate support is not also available to carers.

References

AARONSON, N.K. (1987). *EORTC Protocol 15861: development of a core quality of life questionnaire for use in cancer clinical trials.* Brussels: EORTC Data Center.

AARONSON, N.K., BULLINGER, M. and AHMEDZAI, S. (1988). 'A modular approach to quality-of-life assessment in cancer clinical trials,' in *Recent Results in Cancer Research*, 111: 231–49.

AARONSON, N.K., BAKKER, W., STEWART, A.L. *et al.* (1987). 'Multidimensional approach to the measurement of quality of life in lung cancer clinical trials', in Aaronson, N.K. and Beckmann, J. (Eds), *The Quality of Life of Cancer Patients.* New York: Raven Press, pp. 63–82

AISNER, J. and HANSEN, H.H. (1981). 'Commentary: Current status of chemotherapy for non-small cell lung cancer', in *Cancer Treat. Rep.*, 65: 979–86.

AMERICAN CANCER SOCIETY (1982, July). *Unproven methods of cancer management.* Professional Education Publication No. 3014-PE. New York: American Cancer Society Inc.

AMERICAN PSYCHIATRIC ASSOCIATION (1980). *Diagnostic and statistical manuals of mental disorder*, 3rd ed. Washington, DC: APA.

BLOOM, J.R. (1982). 'Social support, accommodation to stress and adjustment to breast cancer', in *Soc. Sci. Med.*, 16: 1329–38.

BUKBERG, J., PENMAN, D. and HOLLAND, J.C. (1984). 'Depression in hospitalised cancer patients', *Psychosom. Med.*, 436: 199–212.

CANCER RESEARCH CAMPAIGN (1988). *Cancer Factsheets 8.1, 9.1 and 10.1.* London.

CASSILETH, B.R., LUSK, E.J., STROUSE, T.B. and BODENHEIMER, B.J. (1984). 'Contemporary unorthodox treatments in cancer medicine. A study of patients, treatments and practitioners', in *Ann. Int. Med.*, 101: 105–12.

CLARK, A.W. and FALLOWFIELD, L.J. (1986). 'Quality of life measurements in patients with malignant disease: a review', *JRSM*, 79: 165–9.

COATES, A., ABRAHAMS, S., KAYE, S.B. *et al.* (1983). 'On the receiving end—patient perception of the side-effects of cancer chemotherapy', *Eur. J. Ca. Clin. Oncol.*, 19(2): 203–8.

DEROGATIS, L.R., MORROW, G.R. FETTING, J. *et al.* (1983). 'The prevalence of psychiatric disorder among cancer patients', *JAMA*, 249: 751–7.

FALLOWFIELD, L.J. (1988). 'Psychological Complications of Malignant Disease', in *Bailliere's Clinical Oncology*, 2(2) July: 461–78.

FALLOWFIELD, L.J., BAUM, M. and MAGUIRE, G.P. (1986). 'Effects of breast conservation on psychological morbidity associated with diagnosis and treatment of early breast cancer', in *BMJ*, 293: 1331–4.

FOBAIR, P., HOPPE, R.T., BLOOM, J. *et al.* (1986). 'Psychosocial problems among survivors of Hodgkin's disease', in *J. Clin. Oncol.*, 4(5): 805–14.

FORESTER, B.M., KORNFIELD, D.S. and FLEISS, J. (1978). 'Psychiatric aspects of radiotherapy', in *Am. J. Psychiatry*, 135: 960–3.

GRUENDEMANN, B.J. (1965). 'The impact of surgery on body image', in *Nursing Clinics of North America*, 10: 635–43.

HAMILTON, M. (1967). 'Development of a rating scale for primary depressive illness', in *Br. J. Soc. Clin. Psychol.*, 6: 278–96.

HOGBIN, B.J. and FALLOWFIELD, L.J. (1989). 'Getting it taped: the "bad news" consultation in a general surgical outpatients department', *Br. J. Hosp. Med.*, 41: 330–3.

HOUTS, P.S., YASHO, J.M., KAHN, S.B., *et al.* (1986). 'Unmet psychological, social and economic needs of persons with cancer in Pennsylvania', in *Cancer*, 58: 2355–61.

HUGHES, J.E. (1985). 'Depressive illness and lung cancer II: Follow up of inoperable patients', in *Eur. J. Surg. Oncol.*, 11: 21–4.

JONES, S.J. (1981). 'Telling the right patient', *BMJ*, 283: 291–3.

KNOPF, A. (1976). 'Changes in women's opinions about cancer', in *Soc. Sci. Med.*, 10: 191–5.

MAGUIRE, G.P., TAIT, A., BROOKE, M. *et al.* (1980). 'Psychiatric morbidity and physical toxicity associated with adjuvant chemotherapy after mastectomy', *BMJ*, 280: 1179–80.

McINTOSH, J. (1974). 'Processes of communication, information seeking and control associated with cancer. A selective review of the literature', in *Soc. Sci. in Med.*, 8; 167–87.

MOHRER, D., ARTHUR, A.Z. and PATER, J.L. (1984). 'Anticipatory nausea and/or vomiting', in *Cancer Treatment Reps.*, 11: 257–64.

MORRIS, T., GREER, S. and WHITE, P. (1977). 'Psychological and social adjustment to mastectomy: A two year follow-up study', *Cancer*, 40: 2381–7.

MORROW, G.R. and MORROW, C. (1982). 'Behavioural treatment for the anticipatory nausea and vomiting induced by cancer chemotherapy', in *N. Eng. J. Med.*, 307: 1476–80.

MOYNIHAN, C. (1987). 'Testicular cancer: the psychosocial problems of patients and their relatives', in Greer, S. (Ed), 'Psychological aspects of cancer'. *Cancer Surveys*, 6(3): 477–510.

PALMER, B.V., WALSH, G.A., McKENNA, J.A. *et al.* (1980). 'Adjuvant chemotherapy for breast cancer. Side-effects and quality of life', in *BMJ*, 281: 1594–7.

PARSONS, J.A., WEBSTER, J.H. and DOWD, J.E. (1961). 'Evaluation of the placebo effect in the treatment of radiation sickness', in *Acta Radiologica*, 56: 129–40.

PECK, A. and BOLUND, J. (1977). 'Emotional reactions to radiation treatment', in *Cancer*, 40: 180–4.

PENTA, J.S., POSTER, D.S., BRUNO, S. and JACOBS, E.M. (1981). 'Cancer chemotherapy induced nausea and vomiting in adult and paediatric patients', in *Am. Soc. of Clin. Oncol.*, 4: 396.

PETERS-GOLDEN, H. (1982). 'Breast cancer: varied perceptions of social support in the illness experience', in *Soc. Sci. Med.*, 16: 483–91.

PLUMB, M. and HOLLAND, J.C. (1981). 'Comparative studies of psychological function in patients with advanced cancer II', *Psychosom. Med.*, 43: 243–54.

PRIESTMAN, T., BAUM, M., JONES, V. and FORBES, J. (1978). 'Treatment and survival in advanced breast cancer', *BMJ*, 2: 1673–4.

RIEKER, P.P., EDBRIL, S.D. and GARNICK, M.B. (1985). 'Curative testes cancer therapy: psychosocial sequelae', in *J. Clin. Oncol.*, 3: 1117–26.

SCHROVER, L.R. and VON ESCHENBACH, A.C. (1985). 'Sexual and marital relationships after treatment for non-seminomalous testicular cancer', in *J. of Urology*, 25: 251–5.

SILBERFARB, P.M., HOLLAND, J., ANBAR, D. *et al.* (1983). 'Psychological response of patients receiving two drug regimens for lung carcinoma', in *Am. J. Psych.* 140: 110–11.

SILBERFARB, P.M., PHILIBERT, D. and LEVINE, P.M. (1980). 'Psychosocial aspects of neoplastic disease II. Affective and cognitive effects of chemotherapy in cancer patients', in *Am. J. Psychiatry*, 137: 597–601.

SONTAG, S. (1979). *Illness as Metaphor.* London: Alan Lane.

SPIELBERGER, C.D., GORSUCH, R.L. and LUSHENE, R.E. (1968). *State-Trait Anxiety Inventory, Preliminary test manual.* Tallahassee, Florida: Florida State University.

SUGARBAKER, P.H., BAROFSKY, I., ROSENBERG, S.A. and GIANOLA, F.J. (1982). 'Quality of life assessment of patients in extremity sarcoma clinical trials', *Surgery*, 91: 17–23.

TRILLIN, A.S. (1981). 'Of dragons and garden peas: a cancer patient talks to doctors', in *N. Eng. J. Med.*, 304: 699–701.

TWYCROSS, R.G. and GUPPY, D. (1985). 'Prednisolone in terminal breast and bronchogenic cancer', *Practitioner*, 229: 7057–9.

VERRES, R. (1986). *Krebs und Angst.* Berlin-Heidelberg: Springer-Verlag.

WEDDINGTON, W.W., SEGRAVES, K.B. and SIMON, M.A. (1985). 'Psychological outcome of extremity sarcoma survivors undergoing amputation or limb salvage', in *J. Clin. Oncol.*, 3(10): 1393–9.

WEISMAN, A. and WORDEN, W. (1977). *Coping and vulnerability in cancer patients.* Boston: Project Omega.

WING, J.K., COOPER, J.E., SARTORIOUS, N. (1974). *Measurement and Classification of Psychiatric Symptoms.* Cambridge University Press.

ZIGMUND, A.S. and SNAITH, R.P. (1983). 'The Hospital Anxiety and Depression Scale', in *Acta Psychiatr. Scand.*, 67: 361–70.

4   THE QUALITY OF LIFE IN AIDS

Few of the diseases known to man can have caused as much alarm, panic and other acts of ill-informed, irrational behaviour or prejudice as AIDS. It has been likened to the Black Death or pandemic plagues of the Middle Ages (although, as infectious diseases go, AIDS is not particularly contagious). Because primary routes for transmission of the virus are through sexual contact or contaminated needles and syringes, together with the fact that most of the infected people in the West are either homosexuals or drug addicts, we have witnessed an equally virulent, unpleasant epidemic of sanctimonious moralising. Some of the most unedifying aspects of human nature have been displayed by certain individuals who have dismissed the plight and misery of some seriously ill people on the hypocritical grounds that the irresponsible, aberrant behaviour of AIDS victims makes them in some way deserving of their suffering.

AIDS has been dubbed 'the Gay Plague' and it has been claimed to be an expression of the wrath of God towards those with 'abnormal' sexual predilections. A recent book by a lecturer and resource officer of the Christian Medical Fellowship stated:

> Christians do, however, see in the AIDS epidemic the hand of God's judgement on a corrupt society . . . It follows that those who catch it are the victims not only of a lethal virus, but of a society which dresses up as *normal* patterns of behaviour which God condemns.
>
> (Collier, 1987)

Those racially prejudiced members of our society were also given fuel for their unpleasant vendettas when Africa was identified as the probable country of origin of the disease. The

AIDS virus, however, is not prejudiced, and has no particular affinity for homosexuals, heroin users or black Africans, and its steady infiltration into the heterosexual community, together with the tragic infection of haemophiliacs, has led to governmental campaigns, unprecedented in the health education world. The disease has now been reported in 133 different countries (WHO, 1988). One research worker recently stated: 'Any country which has an airport runway long enough to take a Boeing 747 will be likely to have HIV present in the population' (Weber, 1988).

This chapter will look at the effect that AIDS and AIDS related diseases have on the quality of life of patients suffering from the disease and of individuals known to be HIV positive. It will also discuss the difficulties of those who are at high risk of developing the disease and, finally, examine the quality of life experienced by people with the unenviable task of caring for loved ones dying from the disease.

It might be helpful to clear up some confusions that have occurred over nomenclature and provide some definitions. AIDS is an acronym for 'acquired immune deficiency syndrome' and is caused by the human immunodeficiency virus (HIV). The virus invades certain target cells within the body, in particular the T4 lymphocytes controlling the immune system, macrophages which control bacterial infections and microglial brain cells. The latter seem especially vulnerable to the virus, producing distressing neurological and psychiatric dysfunction. Following infection with the virus (often years later), some individuals present with a persistent generalised lymphadenopathy (PGL) in which lymph nodes remain swollen for more than three months. Others with AIDS related complex (ARC) experience malaise, weight loss, fevers, skin rashes, appetite loss, diarrhoea and a generalised lowering of resistance to infections. Many patients with ARC will go on to develop AIDS.

Once the immune system starts to wane following HIV infection, the body becomes extremely susceptible to a wide variety of so-called opportunistic infections and tumours. *Pneumocystis carinii pneumonia*, *Cytomegalovirus* or atypical *Mycobacterial* infections are good examples of opportunistic disease. The protozoal organism *Pneumocystis* is present in most people from childhood, causing no symptoms due to immune surveillance. When the integrity of the immune system is destroyed, for example, by HIV, the *Pneumocystis carinii* organism proliferates, producing an unpleasantly vigorous pneumonia and *Cytomegalovirus* retinitis which causes blindness. Compromised immune surveillance might also permit the development of tumours, such as Kaposi's sarcoma, although the original virus for this, if it is caused by a pathogenic organism, has not yet been identified.

A large number of neurological and psychiatric problems can be identified in patients with HIV invasion of the CNS. Not only is dementia and psychosis common, but such unfortunate individuals may suffer peripheral neuropathy, meningitis, myelitis and encephalopathy, all of which can give rise to fits, paralysis and blindness. There have been reports of AIDS related dementia occurring in patients without any other signs of secondary opportunist infections or tumours.

There is to date no effective curative treatment for the disease other than palliation of some of the unpleasant symptoms. Azidothymidine (AZT, Retrovir, Zovidarine) has been shown to lengthen the survival of patients, but it is too toxic to bone marrow to be used prophylactically in asymptomatic HIV carriers. The quality of well-being scale (QWB) has been used successfully to monitor quality of life and side-effects in clinical trials of AZT (Kaplan *et al.*, 1989).

Problems of the 'Worried Well'

Most sexually active homosexuals, bisexuals and intravenous drug users are, quite naturally, fearful that their high-risk behaviour might result in them contracting the disease. The health education campaigns and media hype have exacerbated this anxiety. Furthermore, witnessing lovers, friends and others dying makes such fears understandable. 'Healthy' anxiety can be useful, however, in initiating positive behavioural changes, such as using clean needles, wearing condoms and limiting sexual partners. It would be a mistake to alleviate fear to a degree that such adaptive behaviours disappeared. What is important, however, is recognising and treating the sort of maladaptive anxiety that results in a neurotic hypervigilance. Some of the 'worried well' develop a crippling and overwhelming conviction that they have symptoms of AIDS. They may engage in obsessive, compulsive behaviours such as constant checking for enlarged lymph nodes or skin lesions, repetitive washing of potential sources of contamination and excessive, persistent ruminations about AIDS. Such morbid preoccupation can lead to constant demands for blood tests which fail to reassure, even when negative; a problem common throughout history, as this quotation reveals:

> . . . here in this unfortunate extreme, if but a pimple appears or any slight ache is felt, they distract themselves with terrible apprehensions . . . And so strongly are they for the most part possessed with this notion that any honest practitioner generally finds it more difficult to cure the imaginary evil than the real one.
>
> Miller (1988) quoting Freind (1727)

Establishing the absence of disease is always difficult, but in the pathologically obsessed it becomes almost impossible. As Dilley (1988) comments:

> Finally, it should be stressed that the patient's symptoms will frequently persist despite the assurance of a negative test. The images of becoming sick with AIDS often persist and serve a self-flagellating, or self-defeating function related to underlying personality issues.

Not surprisingly, these people exhibit clear signs of psychiatric morbidity. Many require psychiatric admission for depression, and suicidal ideation is common. A recent thoughtful paper by Miller (1988) and his colleagues describes some sad case histories, highlighting the disruption caused to ordinary life by AIDS hypochondriasis. Obsessive-compulsive states are well-known as being somewhat resistant to treatment, but Miller *et al.* provide some evidence that cognitive/behavioural psychotherapy can help. Miller *et al.* also point out that there is a historical link with the problems of the current AIDS worried-well and others during previous past epidemics such as syphilis. 'Syphilophobia was first recorded in the medical literature in 1586, over 400 years ago' (MacAlpine 1957). It seems likely that this AIDS phobia will persist until a cure is found and/or another pandemic with both social and life-threatening consequences arises.

QUALITY OF LIFE IN THE HIV POSITIVE

Knowledge that one is seropositive for the AIDS virus can provoke intense psychological suffering. Some writers have suggested that being HIV positive or suffering some signs and symptoms of ARC can be more psychologically distressing than coping with AIDS itself:

> The most common explanation for this finding is that 'life in the Grey Zone', i.e. not knowing what is happening to one's health and constantly living with the spectre of developing AIDS, is more unsettling than actually knowing that one has the full-blown disease.
>
> (Dilley 1988)

Not only does the unfortunate HIV positive individual have to cope with the realisation that he or she faces an almost certain progressive, unpleasant death, but also with an immense psychological burden due to the multifaceted social and moral pressures. In order to protect loved ones from the disease, some may have to 'confess' past misdemeanours or infidelities. In the case of bisexuals or promiscuous hetero-sexuals, this carries the risk of abandonment at a time when stable support within a caring relationship is vital. For homosexuals who have not disclosed their sexual preferences to friends and family, this is also a difficult time. Admission of homosexuality as well as preparing loved ones for the shock that one has a life-threatening disease is sometimes too great an ordeal. Finally, there are enormous financial implications surrounding knowledge that one is HIV positive. It is impossible to get life-insurance, health insurance, endowment mortgages, private pensions and, often, employment. All of these issues may have a profoundly deleterious effect on the quality of life.

Much cant, hypocrisy and illogical thinking has surrounded the debate regarding testing people for the AIDS virus. At one stage it was argued that the testing of any other than the obvious high-risk groups should be discouraged. The reasons given for this suggestion were: 1) that we had no firm evidence that seropositivity invariably led to full-blown AIDS; and 2) that so much stigma and anxiety is aroused by the knowledge that one is seropositive. I have never heard anyone suggest that people suspected of having cancer should not be tested, in case that prevented them from getting a mortgage, or that people who are suspected carriers of infectious diseases such as TB, hepatitis or enteric fever should not be tested in case that prevented them from getting a job.

AIDS is a social problem that potentially affects us all: unless we can help society in general to come to terms with the real plight and moral dilemma facing HIV patients, then we are all at risk. People who are found to be seropositive should be rewarded for their social responsibility and courage with special legislation to protect their jobs and pensions. Compulsory testing is not inconsistent with a desire for the protection of human rights. There should be positive discrimination against those who victimise the HIV positive person. Counselling responsible individuals against being tested denies them the right to protect others.

QUALITY OF LIFE AMONGST AIDS PATIENTS

When symptoms of AIDS finally become manifest, the patient has to contend with an awesome array of assaults on his or her quality of life. Some of the unpleasant physical problems such as the opportunistic infections have already been discussed, but there are other neurological disturbances and a plethora of psychological difficulties.

Neurological disturbances

Approximately 75-80 per cent of patients with AIDs evidence brain pathologies known as HIV encephalitis and HIV encephalopathy (Petito, 1988). These give rise to neurobehavioural changes, sometimes referred to as AIDS dementia complex. Patients start to display cognitive deficits, such as a slowing of learning ability, speech and memory, together with a loss of motor co-ordination. This progresses until the patient demonstrates clear signs of dementia with severe loss of reasoning, speech fluency, amnesia and gross mood swings from extreme agitation and psychosis to apathetic withdrawal. Some also become disorientated and paranoid.

Although such dementia is usually only apparent in terminal

stages of the disease, there are some reports of it being a presenting symptom of AIDS (Navia and Price, 1987, Cummings *et al.*, 1987). A recent report has also shown that as well as the HIV virus producing a primary neuropsychiatric disorder, the virus can be cultured in the CSF of asymptomatic individuals, suggesting that it can infiltrate the central nervous system at a very early stage of the disease (Grant *et al.*, 1988). These authors also conducted a variety of neuropsychological tests, together with nuclear magnetic resonance brain-imaging (NMR) and concluded that AZT is unable to reverse the organic mental disorders provoked by HIV. Thus, there is no effective treatment as yet for the neurological disturbances so common in AIDS.

Psychological distress in AIDS and ARC

Miller and Brown (1988) have discussed the plethora of psychological phenomena associated with HIV infection and disease under six basic headings: 1) shock; 2) fear and anxiety; 3) depression; 4) anger and frustration; 5) guilt; 6) hypochondriasis and obsessive disorders.

1 Shock

Even if patients know themselves to have been at risk from infection, they are often taken by surprise at confirmation of seropositivity and the prospect that they, too, face a premature, unpleasant death. This reaction is similar to the stunned disbelief described by many cancer patients when told their diagnosis.

2 Fear and Anxiety

Although the outcome is ultimately fatal, the uncertainty of the prognosis or likely course of the disease can arouse considerable anxiety and fear. Many AIDS victims have witnessed the disfigurement, disability and death of friends and lovers and are naturally fearful of their own fate. The prospect of dementia and blindness appears to provoke the most anxiety amongst AIDS sufferers. Patients with cancer are often anxious that loved ones will abandon them and that the stigma associated with the diagnosis will produce isolation, social and sexual rejection. The victims of AIDS share similar fears, together with the anxiety that they might infect others or catch a fatal opportunistic infection from friends or loved ones.

3 *Depression*
Depression is common in chronic disease states and AIDS patients are no exception. They experience depression over the various 'losses' sustained as a result of the infection. Not only is there an inevitable loss of health, but they also face a loss of social, occupational and emotional opportunities. Some of the depression associated with AIDS, however, reflects the beginning of a serious organic brain dysfunction. Treatment of AIDS related psychosis may require specialist care from psychiatrists with a particular interest in the management of such patients. The psychiatric needs of the increasing numbers of young people with AIDS has serious consequences for the already underfunded community-based psychiatric services (Fenton, 1988).

4 *Anger and Frustration*
Many patients with AIDS experience anger and frustration at having been 'caught-out' (Miller and Brown, 1988). The 'why me?' syndrome is a common reaction on realising that one has a progressive fatal disease. It is also extremely frustrating to know that one can do little to affect the outcome and that one has to adopt and adapt to new lifestyle restrictions.

5 *Guilt*
A diagnosis of AIDS may reawaken old guilts about being a homosexual or a drug user. Some patients fear that they may also have infected others and experience considerable guilt about this. Other patients, especially those who are very depressed, feel a great deal of self-blame to the extent that they fear that their past misdemeanours have brought about AIDS as a punishment—some sort of divine retribution. This form of guilt has been fuelled by some of the outspoken statements published in the popular press.

6 *Hypochondriasis and Obsessive Disorders*
The obsessional hypervigilant monitoring of the body for new symptoms and signs of AIDS has already been discussed with

reference to the 'worried well'. Patients with AIDS experience all these problems, together with preoccupations about death.

Children with AIDS

The numbers of children with AIDS in this country is still quite small (CDSC, 1988) and, fortunately, since 1987 those haemophiliac children found to be HIV positive as a result of receiving infected blood products have declined appreciably. There are to date (October 1988) 253 children between the ages of 5-14 years known to be HIV positive due to contaminated blood. Interestingly enough, there is some recent research showing that even before being given contaminated blood products, haemophiliacs felt that their chronic handicap was not as great a problem as the prejudice and ignorance of other people (Markova, 1988).

The majority of paediatric AIDS patients (19 children up to August 1988) are infected by their mothers, either during the pregnancy (transplacental or intrapartum) or during the birth (postpartum). Apart from the physical and psychological problems, these children often have a variety of other social problems. An infected mother may not be well enough herself to care for the child and it is always difficult to place children with chronic disease or handicap with foster parents. Many, therefore, are likely to experience only institutional care. Those children still living with their families are likely to suffer a multiplicity of other deprivations, especially if the parents are intravenous drug users who have to resort to other antisocial activities, such as petty crime or prostitution, to support their habit. The quality of life for these children seems unlikely to be anything other than grim. There are fears that many more pregnancies, particularly in Scotland, will be complicated by HIV infection.

QUALITY OF LIFE OF THE CARERS

Caring for a patient with AIDS places a tremendous physical and emotional burden on both health care professionals and relatives, friends and lovers who might look after an AIDS patient at home. Nurses have to develop a wide range of skills which might include: experience with caring for patients with sexually transmitted diseases; experience of barrier nursing and prevention of cross-infection; high-dependency nursing; psychiatric nursing; counselling; and care of the terminally ill. This is extremely demanding for professionals and presents an awesome, sometimes insurmountable challenge for lay-people who may not have had any previous nursing experience at all. Superimpose, upon the physical burden, the emotional toll of watching predominantly young people dying a most unpleasant death and it is not hard to understand why many carers break under the strain.

There has been a considerable amount of research showing that this emotional 'burn-out' produces a deterioration in the sufferer's ability to provide care for AIDS victims, and leads to increased use of drugs and alcohol. If the problems are not recognised and support and help is not given, the carer experiences emotional exhaustion, depersonalisation and a total lack of personal accomplishment or achievement. Those clinicians and nurses who work with cancer patients frequently report feeling emotionally over-extended and exhausted by their work; they feel detached with little empathy for their patients and finally experience a total disillusionment with their own competence (Maslach and Jackson, 1981). There is little reason to suppose that those caring for AIDS patients will fare any better unless some programme of counselling intervention is developed.

Those relatives and friends caring for AIDS patients at home have to confront a variety of other problems which might severely impair their own quality of life. Firstly, there is the undoubted trauma of witnessing a loved one dying. As we have already seen in this chapter, AIDS is disfiguring and disabling. The patients suffer memory losses and some of them develop premature senility. They may go blind and have recurrent bouts of diarrhoea, sickness, bladder infections and skin disease. This can be horrific for those unused to coping with such problems. The lovers of patients dying with AIDS might also be suffering from guilt, especially if they think that they transmitted the virus; or anxiety that they themselves will share a similar fate. Sadly, the homosexual carer might already be trying to cope with the fact of multiple bereavement if other friends have recently become ill and died.

Carers, be they professionals, volunteers or lay people, undoubtedly face a major personal threat to their own psychological stability and quality of life. We must develop and provide appropriate means of support and care for them as well as for the patients.

References

COLLIER, C. (1987). *The 20th Century Plague.* England: Lion Publishing.

COMMUNICABLE DISEASES SURVEILLANCE CENTRE (1988). *Human Immunodeficiency Virus.* Colindale, London.

CUMMINGS, M.A., CUMMINGS, K.L., RAPAPORT, M.H. *et al.* (1987). 'Acquired immune deficiency syndrome (AIDS) presenting as schizophrenia', in *Western Journal of Medicine,* 146: 615.

DILLEY, J.W. (1988). 'Psychiatric sequelae of HIV', in: Paine, L. (Ed), *AIDS: Psychiatric and Psychological Perspectives.* London: Croom Helm.

FENTON, T.W. (1988). 'Psychiatric aspects of HIV infection: implications for the UK', in *J. Roy. Coll. of Phys. of London,* 22(3): 145–8.

FREIND, J. (1727) *The History of Physick*, 2nd Ed, Part 2. London: Walthoe.

GRANT, I., HAMPTON ATKINSON, J., HESSELINK, J.R. *et al.* (1988). 'Human immunodeficiency virus-associated neurobehavioural disorder', in *J. Roy. Coll. Physicians of London,* 22(3): 149–57.

KAPLAN, R.M., ANDERSON, J.P., WU, A.W., *et al.* (1989). 'The quality of well-being scale. Applications in AIDS, Cystic Fibrosis and Arthritis', in *Medical Care,* 23(3): 27–43.

MACALPINE, I. (1957). 'Syphilophobia: a psychiatric study', in *British Journal of Venereal Diseases,* 33: 92.

MARKOVA, I. (1988). 'Haemophiliacs expect prejudice', in *The Psychologist,* 1(2): 49.

MASLACH, C. and JACKSON, S.E. (1981). *The Maslach Burnout Inventory.* Palo Alto, CA: Consulting Psychologists Press.

MILLER, D., ACTON, T. and HEDGE, B. (1988). 'The worried well: their identification and management', in *J. R. Coll. Physicians of London,* 22(3): 158–65.

MILLER, D. and BROWN, B. (1988). 'Developing the role of clinical psychology in the context of AIDS', in *The Psychologist: Bulletin of the British Psychological Society*, 2: 63-6.

NAVIA, B.A. and PRICE, R.W. (1987). 'The acquired immunodeficiency syndrome dementia complex as the presenting or sole manifestation of human immunodeficiency virus infection', in *Archives of Neurology*, 44: 65-9.

PETITO, C.K. (1988). 'Review of central nervous system pathology in human immunodeficiency virus infection', in *Annals of Neurology*, 23(suppl): 527-33.

WEBER, J. (1988). 'The Biology of HIV', in Paine, L. (Ed), *AIDS: Psychiatric and Psychosocial Perspective*. London: Croom Helm, pp. 1-11.

WHO (1988). *World Health Organisation press release.*

5 THE QUALITY OF LIFE IN CARDIOVASCULAR DISEASE

Ischaemic heart disease kills approximately 193,000 people annually in England and Wales and is the greatest killer of all the diseases known to Western man. Coronary artery disease due to atherosclerosis is responsible for most of these deaths (163,104 in 1985), and approximately 500,000 new cases are diagnosed each year. Although there are noticeable regional variations, 30 per cent of all deaths in men and 22 per cent in women in England and Wales are due to ischaemic heart disease. Cerebrovascular accidents (CVAs), or strokes which occur as a result of similar degenerative processes in the arteries of the brain, are another major cause of disability and death, killing 67,000 people in England alone in 1980 (Fry et al., 1984).

Due to the alarming prevalence of cardiovascular disease and the millions of pounds spent annually attempting to treat it, there is an increasing interest in the measurement of quality of life as an assessment of the efficacy of different therapies.

In view of the enormity of the subject, I have chosen to cover four main topics in this chapter.

Firstly, I shall look at the psychological impact of chronic heart disease, in particular angina and myocardial infarction, and include a brief discussion of some of the literature concerning quality of life after open heart surgery. This will be followed with a description of the large number of physical, psychological and social consequences that cerebrovascular accidents have for patients and their families. Finally, I shall consider the quality of life during long-term hypertensive therapy which aims to control high blood pressure, thereby reducing the risk of coronary heart disease and stroke.

Quality of Life with Angina and Following Mycocardial Infarction (Heart Attack)

In ischaemic heart disease the coronary arteries are narrowed by fatty deposits (atheroma). The build-up of plaque may become large enough completely to block or thrombose the artery which leads to death of the heart muscle—a myocardial infarction. Although myocardial infarctions may occur suddenly, with little warning, many people will have experienced bouts of angina for some time. Angina is described as a tight, crushing pain in the chest, which often radiates up into the neck, and is accompanied by tachycardia (palpitations). It is usually brought on by exertion, a heavy meal or extreme emotion. Apart from the pain, it is also very frightening, as most people are well aware that such symptoms may herald a heart attack or even a cardiac arrest and death. Consequently, anxiety about the future, especially fears of sudden death, may overwhelm some patients.

Although angina can be treated and controlled satisfactorily for many years with appropriate drugs and/or surgery, it often requires quite dramatic changes of lifestyle. Frequently the most susceptible patients are obese, unfit smokers and they may also have stressful, sedentary occupations together with a family history of heart disease. Behavioural changes such as dieting, exercise and giving up smoking are important, but this may be problematic for some, due to their working conditions and to family dynamics. Encouraging major behavioural changes is also difficult due to the high prevalence of certain personality factors amongst susceptible patients. This is a controversial issue, but many individuals with coronary heart disease evidence characteristic personality traits, the so-called Type A Behaviour Pattern. The primary manifestations of Type A personality are obsessional time urgency, a high need for achievement and excessive ambition, intolerance and impatience, over-involvement with work and sometimes overt hostility and aggression. One rigorous prospective epidemiological project, the Western Collaborative Group Study, screened 3,154 males for Type A Behaviour. The study subjects were all healthy at the initial assessment, but follow-up investigations for eight and a half years showed that those men with Type A personalities had almost twice the incidence of coronary heart disease over the study period (Rosenman *et al.*, 1975).

There are several different methods of measuring Type A Behaviour, but the two most commonly used techniques are the structured interview (Rosenman *et al.*, 1975) and the Jenkins Activity Survey (Jenkins, 1979). As neither of these tests is, strictly speaking, a quality of life instrument, I shall not describe them in any detail, but they are important measures of the efficacy of behaviour modification programmes (Chesney *et al.*, 1981). These programmes aim to help patients alter those traits and behaviour patterns which might predispose them to attacks of angina or myocardial infarction. The maintenance of a different lifestyle following a successful behavioural modification programme produces changes in the quality of life, especially if a change of employment is involved. As these programmes help individuals to manage their hostility, impatience and driving ambition, they can make patients easier to live with, thus improving the quality of life of other family members.

Following a diagnosis of coronary heart disease, some patients report that their spouses or partners become over-protective and controlling about diet, exercise, rest or sexual activities, all of which can severely impair the relationship. Adapting to potentially life-threatening illness is demanding for the family as well as the patient, and I shall discuss this problem later in the chapter.

Drug Therapy

Beta-blockers belong to one of the drug groups commonly used to treat angina. They work by reducing the heart rate and arterial pressure and permitting more time for blood flow in the coronary arteries. Whilst beta-blockers are effective in controlling the pain and thus improving quality of life, this relief is not arrived at without certain costs and side-effects; in particular insomnia, nightmares, tiredness, bronchoconstriction and impotence. There is also some evidence that beta-blockers produce cognitive impairment (Lichter *et al.*, 1984), especially memory deficits.

Another common pharmacological means of managing angina is with nitrates, such as glyceryl trinitrate (GTN).

Taken either in tablet or spray form, this drug usually brings about rapid relief of pain. The drugs do produce severe headaches in some patients, together with flushing and sometimes fainting due to hypotension (low blood pressure). Some authors have described the social problems that taking nitroglycerin can provoke. Slaby and Glicksman (1985) report the case of a patient with angina who always took the medication surreptitiously, as he recognised that overtly taking the drug made other people very anxious and uncomfortable: 'I can clear a room just by taking that bottle out and very obviously sticking one of these under my tongue.'

Recently, the use of long-acting nitrates, delivered over 24-hour periods via self-adhesive skin patches, has been advocated and there have been claims that this mode of drug administration is acceptable to most patients. Transdermal patches would, of course, overcome the social problems associated with taking GTN sublingually to obtain relief from angina. However, a double-blind randomised clinical trial of transdermal glyceryl trinitrate or placebo in 427 men with stable angina showed that continuous use of GTN administered in this way failed to prevent angina attacks and furthermore affected quality of life (Fletcher *et al.*, 1988). Patients with the active drug skin-patches reported many more headaches than those with the placebo, and these were often severe enough for them to withdraw from the trial. Assessment of quality of life using the Sickness Impact Profile (SIP) (see Chapter 2) showed a decline in social interaction when patients were receiving the active drug patch. This psychosocial disruption might have been due to the increase in headaches. The inclusion of a quality of life measure in this study provided important evaluation data and demonstrates the usefulness of including such assessments alongside the more traditional parameters of benefit.

Many patients feel anxious that a patient taking GTN will have a heart attack there and then before their eyes, and this leads to avoidance of the unfortunate patient. Such reactions are, of course, profoundly upsetting for an individual who wants to lead a normal life, but who is actually dependent on others taking prompt action should he or she need assistance. In contrast, other patients have also described their irritation at the excessive solicitude displayed by their family members or friends; for example a visit to the lavatory is frequently interrupted by people knocking on the door to enquire if the occupant is still all right!

Surgery

Those patients who have localised narrowing of the main coronary arteries may benefit from surgery, either coronary artery bypass grafting (CABG) or coronary angioplasty. The relative merits and medical indications for these procedures are beyond the scope of this book, but it is clear that quality of life assessment plays an important part in the decision to opt for surgical management of CHD, and that quality of life measures must form a major part of the evaluation of the outcome of surgery. Despite earlier hopes that surgery would improve the life expectancy of patients with angina, controlled clinical trials such as the Coronary Artery Surgery Study (CASS) in 1983 have been disappointing. In comparison with medical management, no demonstrable survival advantages have been shown with surgery other than in a small subset of patients. The operative mortality risk from CABG varies and depends on such things as sex (women suffer four times the operative mortality and perioperative infarction rates of men), which vessels are involved, and whether the patient has stable or unstable angina.

For the majority of patients the risk of up to ten per cent of immediate death from surgery cannot be justified if the sole measure of efficacy is improvement in life expectancy. Quality of life considerations are therefore imperative and, what is more, reveal a clear benefit to patients from surgical intervention. A review of the research literature reporting the outcome of 14 different controlled clinical trials showed that coronary artery bypass grafting conveys a 25-40 per cent better chance that patients will be free from angina than that obtained from medical treatment (Wortman and Yeaton, 1985). Relief of pain permits patients to engage in more activities of daily living, such as a return to work and leisure pursuits.

One quality of life measure that seems appropriate for evaluating outcome following CABG is the SIP, which has already been mentioned in this section as the method used to assess the merits of continuous GTN therapy using skin patches. Vandenburg (1988) has shown that the SIP discriminates well between angina patients and healthy controls. He reported that the 50 angina patients studied showed impairment in all 12 categories when compared with 50 matched controls, but that these impairments were especially marked in the work and recreation categories. Most studies show that post-surgery freedom from angina permits 50 to 75 per cent of patients to return to work. However, Pugsley and Treasure (1987) point out, in a readable and succinct paper describing the techniques and pros and cons of the surgical approach to angina, that many patients who are physically capable of work fail to return for a variety of reasons. Some individuals may be of an age where early retirement was feasible; others who were without jobs for six months prior to surgery are unlikely to work again, and manual workers with heavy physical work loads seem to remain unemployed, giving poor health as a reason for continued unemployment. This highlights the necessity for using several different measures of quality of life, not just 'return to work', if error in interpreting the outcome of various therapies is to be avoided.

Myocardial Infarction

Anxiety and depression are common sequelae to a sudden unexpected life-threatening illness, such as myocardial infarction. Lloyd and Cawley (1983) reported that a fifth of the patients whom they studied a week after an acute myocardial infarction had significant adjustment disorders and psychological symptoms. However, these were transitory symptoms which had disappeared when the patients were reassessed four months later.

Although these data show that the initial phase of recovery from myocardial infarction disrupts psychological and social functioning for a limited period, a significant minority of patients experience unrelenting periods of psychosocial morbidity and marital stress. Finlayson and McEwan (1977) studied the psychosocial impact of myocardial infarction on 76 married men four years after their first infarction. Twelve per cent of their sample had been unable to resume a stable pattern of social activity with friends, and almost half (49 per cent) experienced a decrease in their social lives in comparison with that enjoyed prior to the infarction. In another study, Mayou *et al.* (1978) interviewed 100 patients on three occasions, on admission, at two months and at 12 months following their first myocardial infarction. They reported rather different findings from those of Lloyd and Cawley: leisure pursuits had dramatically altered in 30 per cent of the patients and another 36 per cent had not resumed all their previous activities. Mayou also found high levels of psychiatric morbidity, with 64 per cent of patients showing anxiety, depression and other adjustment disorders. One important point made by Mayou (1984) was that high initial distress was unremitting. Thus a thorough psychiatric assessment of patients at an early stage might help identify those at risk from experiencing protracted social disability and psychiatric morbidity.

The impact that myocardial infarction has on the quality of life of spouses of victims is also worthy of some consideration, as they too have a considerable amount of adaptation and adjustment to make on many fronts. Mayou reported that any affective disorders among patients were invariably evident in their spouses, as was social dysfunction. Almost 50 per cent of the couples interviewed reported a reduction in sexual activity since the patient's myocardial infarction, although for some this was welcomed. Interestingly, almost a quarter of the spouses perceived an improvement in the quality of their marriages after the patients' illness, with more evidence of tolerance and consideration. Some wives did admit that they were forced to avoid confrontation and quarrels for fear of precipitating another heart attack. Resentment and irritation about over-protectiveness was expressed by 18 per cent of the men, together with feelings of humiliation and frustration in 25 per cent of the sample about their different role within the family, watching their wives doing 'men's jobs'.

Finlayson and McEwan (1977) suggest that assessment of the full implications of myocardial infarction in terms of a patient's recovery and rehabilitation may take several years. Thus indicators of successful outcome should involve several measures of different aspects of a patient's lifestyle taken at different points in time. Whilst return to work and freedom from chest pain are important indices of outcome, emotional and social dysfunction need to be considered as well. Some patients have little option but to return to work, especially if they have jobs without the protection of pension rights when early retirement due to ill-health is taken. Others may return to rather different paid employment and suffer a loss of both status and income. Initially the pleasure at having survived a heart attack and the sense of well-being might be of maximal importance to an individual, but changed status might have a profoundly depressing effect later on. One study by Byrne (1982) followed up male survivors of a myocardial infarction (mean age 54 years) at eight months and again at 24 months. At eight months 85 per cent of the sample had returned to paid employment, but two years post infarction only 65 per cent were still working. Byrne suggests that some patients might return to work prematurely against medical advice and then have to change jobs or take further sick leave, none of which enhances self-esteem.

It is interesting to note that most studies show that more white collar workers return to work than blue collar workers, irrespective of the severity of the myocardial infarction. Byrne (1980) also reported that those patients in blue collar occupations revealed significantly more anxiety than those in white collar occupations, presumably due to fears that their manual activities might predispose them to further myocardial infarction, although it is possible that they also had more financial worries.

It is clear that any measurement of the quality of life following treatments for either angina or myocardial infarction must consider parameters such as family relationships, work and leisure pursuits, psychiatric morbidity and sexual activity, as well as freedom from pain. Heart disease affects all these areas of daily living and assessment of them is just as important as measures of physical functioning.

Cerebrovascular Disease
Cerebrovascular accidents (CVA) account for 67,000 deaths annually in England. The most common form of CVA is haemorrhage from a diseased blood vessel, particularly in the elderly—especially those with hypertension. The incidence and mortality from CVA increases with age, but at least 25 per

cent of CVA victims are under the age of 65 and therefore still in full-time employment.

Anyone who survives the initial trauma of a stroke will suffer some impairment to their physical, social, cognitive and emotional functioning. The degree of disability varies enormously, from minor dysfunction to major impairment involving paralysis, dysarthria and a severe alteration of mood and cognitive ability. Such problems often involve the patient in a quite radical adjustment to lifestyle. It also means considerable change for the family, friends and work associates of an affected individual. Furthermore, outcome is often uncertain: some patients do regain a certain amount of function which is sustained until the end of their lives, whereas other remain permanently disabled and may indeed suffer further strokes or die. The quality of life following CVA may be dependent on factors within biological, psychological and social domains and seems related also to an individual's premorbid level of functioning in each of those domains.

Neimi *et al.* (1988) looked at the quality of life in 46 stroke survivors under the age of 65, four years after their first stroke. They developed a comprehensive questionnaire that covered four areas of daily living: work, leisure, domestic activities and family relationships (see Table 22). Although patients were fit enough to have been discharged from hospital, the quality of life had not been restored to its prestroke level in 83 per cent of those studied. Depression, paresis, the location of the lesion and co-ordination difficulties were all highly correlated with a deterioration in quality of life, as were an inability to return to work and dependence on others for assistance with daily life.

Depression is a very common feature following CVA. Figures vary according to the assessment schedules used and variables such as the age of the patient, degree of handicap and length of time since the stroke, but most studies find that at least one half of hospitalised stroke victims and one third of all other stroke patient populations are depressed (Starkstein *et al.*, 1988). Ahlsiö *et al.* (1984) used a visual analogue scale to assess quality of life and noted that depression played a major role in patients' evaluation of their quality of life. Two years post-stroke, 77 per cent of patients had a deterioration of quality of life. One study by Robinson and Szetela (1981)

TABLE 22

Quality of Life After Stroke
Domains of Life and Sample Questions in Each Domain

Working Conditions	Activities at home	Family relationships including close personal relationships and sexual patterns	Leisure time activities in and outside home
Employment Work satisfaction	Participation in preparation of meals	Participation in family decision-making (major investments, loans, and so on)	Participation or interest in:
Attitudes of fellow workers toward you	If living alone, preparation of meals	If living alone, independent decision-making (major investments, loans, and so on)	Outdoor activities (walking, camping, swimming, games, etc.)
Attitude of supervisors toward you	Participation in cleaning		Family festivities or other occasions arranged by relatives
Own attitudes toward fellow workers	If living alone, cleaning		Parties arranged by friends or acquaintances
Own attitudes towards supervisors	Participation in laundry		Going dancing
	If living alone, laundry		Going to movies, theaters, concerts, etc

reported that 61 per cent of their patients were clinically depressed. This study was particularly interesting because only patients who had suffered a cerebrovascular accident in the left hemisphere were tested. The integrity of the left hemisphere is necessary for speech production in 95 per cent of right-handed people and in 70 per cent of left-handers. Thus, many of these patients had severe speech deficits (dysarthria and/or aphasia) following their strokes and this appeared to have contributed to a large amount of their depression (Robinson and Benson, 1981).

Starkstein et al. (1988) have suggested that patients who experience cortical lesions rather than subcortical or posterior circulation strokes, suffer irreversible damage to areas thought to be important parts of ascending biogenic amine pathways which profoundly influence mood state. Depression which fails to recover with time is seen therefore more frequently in patients who have suffered left frontal cortical or basal ganglia lesions.

Following the acute phase of a CVA, most patients are discharged from hospital to the care of relatives. As CVA predominantly affects people in the latter part of their lives, this often means that another elderly person might have to cope with their care, largely unsupported. The level of dependence of stroke victims sometimes proves to be an intolerable burden on their spouses. Two studies (Kinsella and Duffy, 1979; Brockenhurst et al., 1981) have reported an increase in health problems and depressive illness amongst the families of stroke victims. In another interesting report, Wade et al. (1986) found that even those carers looking after patients with little obvious mental and physical disability suffer distress and depression with increasing incidence as time goes by. Thus the quality of life for those left with primary responsibility for the care of patients seems to decline, irrespective of the level of physical and mental functioning, and therefore merits attention.

Provision of support in terms of home helps, adaptation of equipment to assist with mobility, toileting and bathing, can all greatly enhance the ability of relatives to care for disabled patients more adequately and improve the quality of life, but this alone is insufficient. As a professor of geriatric medicine (MacLennan, 1988) points out in a recent thoughtful review:

The various services on offer suggest that a mechanical approach will provide a solution to the problems of stroke families. It will not. Emotional relationships are often at least as important as physical incapacity in determining a satisfactory adjustment to stroke. It is probable therefore that the clinical psychologist as well as the doctor, nurse and rehabilitationist will have a major role in the house care of stroke families.

The attitude of the family to the stroke victim seems to influence the rehabilitation outcome. Adler *et al.* (1969) studied 5,486 Israeli stroke patients. One hundred and twenty patients and their families had a more comprehensive assessment of the family relationship and patients were rated using an activities of daily living schedule. Positive family attitudes, such as wishing the patient to be at home rather than in hospital, encouraging independence, not regarding the patient as a burden and wanting the patient to become more active, correlated highly with a good rehabilitative outcome. Those families who pitied the stroke victim and viewed him or her as a hopeless, helpless burden, did not assist his recovery.

Hypertension

One method of reducing the risk of both CVA and CHD is to control blood pressure. However, the point at which a high blood pressure increases risk of CHD and CVA is a controversial issue. The literature is full of debates about the value of giving anti-hypertensive therapy to middle-aged people suffering from mild hypertension, or to those who are asymptomatic. If anti-hypertensives had no side-effects there would probably be no argument, but such drugs produce a catalogue of problems which diminish quality of life sufficiently for patients to abandon taking them, thus risking a CVA or heart attack. One study by Sackett and Haynes (1976), suggests that as many as 50 per cent of hypertensive patients cease taking their prescribed drugs after only six months. It is not difficult to understand why a patient might feel that on balance a dry mouth, nausea, headache, extreme fatigue and impotence constituted a diminution in the quality of life of far greater magnitude than the anxiety that his blood pressure, if uncontrolled, might provoke a stroke or heart attack. Light (1980) has commented on the other behavioural side-effects associated with specific anti-hypertensive drugs. More recently Jachuck *et al.* (1982) reported that approximately two thirds of patients prescribed anti-hypertensive drugs felt that the therapy was exerting an adverse effect on their quality of life despite their physician's perception of effective control of blood pressure.

Fortunately, there is an increasing number of clinical trials examining different therapeutic options, not only in terms of physical morbidity and mortality, but also measuring outcome in terms of the impact on various quality of life variables. However, side-effects provoke a large number of patients to withdraw from studies—for example, the (1981) MRC trial of mild hypertension therapy found that over the five-year study period ten per cent of patients withdrew, due to adverse side-effects, the primary complaints being impotence, lethargy, gout, nausea, dizziness and headache. Furthermore, this study showed no reduction in mortality and only a minimal reduction in the number of strokes.

Many patients taking anti-hypertensives are depressed (although, as Fletcher *et al.* (1987) have pointed out, mere labelling of an essentially asymptomatic patient as hypertensive might influence psychological well-being). There is also some evidence that hypertensive patients, whether treated or not, experience measurable impairments to both memory and learning ability (Solomon *et al.*, 1983; Franchesci, 1982).

Effect on quality of life may be to some extent dependent on age, sex and cultural background. A Dutch study of 420 hypertension patients showed that symptom distress was reported more frequently in the 50-59 age group than in younger (under 50) and older (over 60) patients. Furthermore, the older patients scored less on depression and inadequacy scales than other groups (Curb *et al.*, 1985). Perhaps these results are not all that surprising, as Fletcher *et al.* comment that the older hypertensive patients might well 'have an increased expectation of chronic disease, or a modified pharmacokinetic response to drugs'. Another interesting finding in the Dutch study was that the female patients had higher somatic and psychiatric dysfunction than the men, irrespective of age.

The problems encountered by patients suffering from cardio- or cerebrovascular disease are legion, and this chapter has merely outlined some of the ways in which quality of life is threatened. Successful coping with a wide variety of psychosocial crises requires patients to find and develop adaptive strategies. They may have to learn to live with pain, breathlessness and incapacitation; they might have to cope with repeated visits to hospital and constant monitoring of treatment procedures. Within this framework of dependence on health professionals, family and drugs, they have to find some means of self-assertion and sense of mastery and competence. They may find sustaining relationships with family, friends and work colleagues extremely difficult. Finally, to lead a well-adjusted life patients have to learn how to manage an uncertain future.

Sensible quality of life assessment may help identify those patients in need of extra support, be that physical help and/or counselling. It may also play a vital part in evaluating the efficacy of new treatments for the large number of cardio- and cerebro-vascular diseases that claim so many lives in the western world.

References

ADLER, E., ADLER, C., MAGORA, A. *et al.* (1969). *Stroke in Israel 1957-1961. Epidemiological, clinical, rehabilitation and psychosocial aspects.* Jerusalem: Polypress Ltd.

AHLSIÖ, B., BRITTON, M., MURRAY, V. *et al.* (1984). 'Disablement and quality of life after stroke', in *Stroke*, 15: 886–90.

BROCKENHURST, J.C., MORRIS, P., ANDREWS, K. *et al.* (1981). 'Social effects of stroke', in *Sco. Sci. Med.*, 15: 35–9.

BYRNE, D.G. (1980). 'Effects of social context on psychological responses to survived myocardial infarction', in *Int. J. of Psych. in Med.*, 10: 23–31.

BYRNE, D.G. (1981). 'Type A behaviour, life events and myocardial infarction: independent or related risk factors?' in *Br. J. Med. Psych.*, 54: 371–7.

BYRNE, D.G. (1982). 'Psychological response to illness and outcome after survived myocardial infarction: A long-term follow-up', *J. of Psych. Res.*, 26: 105–12.

CASS. Principal Investigators and their Associates (1983). 'Coronary artery surgery study (CASS): a randomised trial of coronary artery bypass survival data', in *Circulation*, 68: 939–50.

CHESNEY, M.A., EAGLESTON, J.R. and ROSENMAN, R.H. (1981). 'Type A Behaviour: Assessment and Intervention', in Prokop, C.K. and Bradley, L.A. (Eds), *Medical Psychology*. New York: Academic Press.

CURB, J.D., BORTIANI, N.O., BLASZKANSKI, T.P. *et al.* (1985). 'Long-term surveillance for adverse effects of hypertensive drugs', in *JAMA*, 253: 3263–8.

FINLAYSON, A. and MCEWEN, J. (1977). *Coronary Heart Disease and Patterns of Living*. London: Croom Helm.

FLETCHER, A.E., HUNT, B.M. and BULPITT, C.J. (1987). 'Evaluation of quality of life in clinical trials of cardiovascular disease', in *J. Chron. Dis.*, 40(6): 557–66.

FLETCHER, A.E., MCLOONE, P. and BULPITT, C. (1988). 'Quality of life on angina therapy: a randomised controlled trial of transdermal glyceryl trinitrate against placebo', in *Lancet*, (i) 4–7.

FRANCHESCI, M., TANCREDI, A. SMIRNE, S. *et al.* (1982). 'Cognitive processes in hypertension', in *Hypertension*, 31: 226–9.

FRY, J., BROOKS, D., and MCCOLL, I. (1984). *NHS Data Book*. Lancaster: MTP.

JACHUCK, S.J., BRIERLEY, H., JACHUCK, S. and WILLCOX, P.M. (1982). 'The effect of hypotensive drugs on the quality of life', in *J. Roy. Coll. Gen. Practitioners*, 32: 103–5.

JENKINS, D.C., ZYZANSKI, S.J. and ROSENMAN, R.H. (1979). *Jenkins Activity Survey Manual (Form C)*. New York: The Psychological Corporation.

KINSELLA, G.J. and DUFFY, F. (1979). 'Psychosocial readjustment in the spouses of aphasic patients', in *Scand. J. Rehab. Med.*, 11: 129–132.

LICHTER, I., RICHARDSON, P.J. and WYKE, M.A. (1984). 'Differential effects of atenolol and enalapril on tests of memory during treatment for essential hypertension', in *J. Hypertens.*, 2: 560.

LIGHT, K.C. (1980). 'Antihypertensive drugs and behavioural performance', in Elias, M.F. and Streeton, D.H.P. (Eds), *Hypertension and Cognitive Processes*, Maine: Beech Hill Publishing Company, p. 120.

LLOYD, G.G. and CAWLEY, R.H. (1983). 'Distress or illness? A study of psychological symptoms after myocardial infarction', in *Br. J. Psychiatry*, 142: 120–5.

MacLennan, W.J. (1988). 'Stroke management care for stroke patients: community and hospital', in *Geriatric Med.* 35–41.

Mayou, R., Foster, A. and Williamson, B. (1978). 'Psychosocial adjustment in patients one year after myocardial infarction', in *J. Psychosom. Res.*, 22: 447–53.

Mayou, R. (1979). 'The course and determinants of reactions to myocardial infarction', in *Br. J. Psychiatry*, 134: 588–94.

Mayou, R. (1984). 'Prediction of emotional and social outcome after a heart attack', in *J. of Psych. Res.*, 28: 17–25.

Medical Research Council Working Party On Mild To Moderate Hypertension. (1981). 'Adverse reactions to bendrofluazide and propranolol for the treatment of mild hypertension', in *Lancet*, ii: 539–43.

Neimi, M.L., Laarksonen, R., Kotila, M. and Waltimo, O. (1988). 'The quality of life four years after stroke', in *Stroke* 19(9): 1101–7.

Pugsley, W.N. and Treasure, T. (1987). 'The Surgical Approach', in Julian, D.G. (Ed), *Ischaemic Heart Disease.* Surrey: Update, Siebart Publications Ltd.

Robinson, R. and Benson, D.R. (1981). 'Depression in aphasic patients: Frequency, severity and clinical-pathological correlations', in *Brain and Language*, 14: 282–91.

Robinson, R.G. and Szetela, B. (1981). 'Mood change following left hemispheric brain injury', in *Annals of Neurology*, 9: 447–53.

Rosenman, R.H., Brand, R.J., Jenkins, C.D. *et al.* (1975). 'Coronary heart disease in the western collaborative group study', in *JAMA*, 233: 872–7.

Sackett, D.L. and Haynes, R.B. (1976). *Compliance with therapeutic regimens.* Baltimore: Johns Hopkins University Press, p. 175.

Slaby, A.E. and Glicksman, A.S. (1985). *Adapting to Life-threatening Illness.* New York: Praeger Publishers.

Solomon, S., Hotchkiss, E., Saravay, S.M. *et al.* (1983). 'Impairment of memory function by hypertensive medication', in *Arch. Gen. Psych.*, 40: 1109–12.

STARKSTEIN, S.E., ROBINSON, R.G. and PRICE, T.R. (1988). 'Comparison of spontaneously recovered versus non-recovered patients with post-stroke depression', in *Stroke*, 19(12): 1491–6.

VANDENBURG, M.J. (1988). 'Measuring quality of life in patients with angina', in Walker, S.R. and Rosser, R.M. (Eds), *Quality of Life: Assessment and Application*. London: Ciba Foundation.

WADE, D.T., LEGH-SMITH, J. and HEWER, R.L. (1986). 'Effects of living with and looking after survivors of a stroke', in *BMJ*, 293: 418–20.

WORTMAN, P.M. and YEATON, W.H. (1985). 'Cumulating quality of life results in controlled trials of coronary artery bypass graft surveys', in *Controlled Clinical Trials*, 6: 289–305.

6 THE QUALITY OF LIFE IN ARTHRITIS

All the diseases with which I have dealt in previous chapters affect not only the *quality* of sufferers' lives, they may also threaten life itself. There are, however, many other chronic, non-fatal disease states, for example arthritis, which seriously compromise the quality of life and sense of well-being of patients.

Arthritis is a very common chronic disease in the western world which, according to the British Arthritis and Rheumatism Council for Research, affects at least one in ten people in Britain to a major or minor degree. Although it is a problem that most people associate with the elderly, there are in fact more than 12,000 juvenile rheumatoid arthritis sufferers in this country and the vast majority of rheumatoid arthritis patients are between the ages of 25 and 55 years. The incidence of the disease is three times greater amongst women than in men and there appears to be a familial tendency.

Arthritis takes many forms and the amount of pain, disablement and consequent treatment depends to a certain extent on the type of arthritis. In this chapter I shall discuss the quality of life in two broad categories of arthritic disease: rheumatoid arthritis (RA) and osteoarthritis (OA). A very basic distinction between the two is that in RA the synovial membrane surrounding the joint becomes inflamed (synovitis) and in OA the joint cartilage degenerates. Both produce warm, swollen and tender joints, making movement difficult and painful, but with RA there is a characteristic early morning stiffness and in OA mobility tends to worsen later in the day.

Rheumatoid Arthritis
The onset of RA is usually insidious, with patients describing a period of having felt generally unwell—a loss of energy, perhaps some weight loss, insomnia and, importantly, swelling

and pain in one or more joints for at least six weeks. Patients usually notice that a period of immobility tends to worsen the pain and stiffness, especially following a night's sleep. Other diagnostic features are the identification of rheumatoid factor in the blood and rheumatoid nodules over bony prominences such as the elbows. In contrast to OA, where there may be unilateral joint swelling, RA usually affects both sides of the body, giving rise to symmetrical joint swelling. The wrists and knuckles are nearly always involved, together with the knees, but any joint may be affected. Because of the difficulty of movement, the muscles supplying the affected joints may become wasted. The appearance of the hands of an RA sufferer with advanced chronic disease is characteristic, with swollen joints (especially those at the base of the hand) wasted muscles and often dislocated fingers. At this stage, quite simple tasks of everyday life, such as hair brushing, dressing or unscrewing a jar, may become excruciatingly painful or impossible.

Osteoarthritis

This is not primarily an inflammatory disorder, as is RA, but tends to be the end result of degenerative changes in the cartilage, with secondary changes occurring around and/or in the affected joints. Particularly affected are the weight-bearing joints, especially the hips and knees.

This progressive cartilage loss seems to be associated with other features, primarily the formation of bony outgrowths around the ends of finger joints, called Heberden's nodes. Although osteoarthritis is associated with old age, promoting the hypothesis that it is a gradual mechanical 'wearing-out' of the joints, there is evidence that it might also have a biochemical cause. A detailed description of the controversy surrounding the aetiology of OA is beyond the range of this book, but some protagonists of the degenerative hypothesis have suggested that osteoarthritis is universal and would be seen in all of us if we lived long enough. Lawrence (1977), for example, suggested that 52 per cent of all adults in Britain have at least one joint showing the degenerative changes of OA, and it has been estimated that 44 per cent of all physical disability in the elderly can be attributed to arthritis (Dorevitch, 1988). Others have pointed out that it is a mistake to suggest that the disease is 'degenerative' just because it occurs in the elderly (Huskisson, 1985).

The pattern of the disease, in terms of which joints are involved, can be rather different, which might also suggest different causal factors. The OA seen in the knee joint of a youngish man with a history of injury seems qualitatively different from the elderly lady with disease in the finger joints of both hands. As in RA, women seem to suffer more than men from OA. They tend to be over 50, with a family history of the disease, and appear to experience problems primarily in the distal interphalangeal joints of the hands. Men more commonly have OA confined to one hip, with one in five of males in the North of England over the age of 55 years affected in this way. Support for the idea that trauma produces arthritic changes came from the observation that cotton spinners and weavers had a high incidence of Heberden's nodes due to the repetitive daily trauma inflicted by their work. Contrary to popular belief, there is little evidence that overuse of a joint in, for example, the knees or shoulders of sportsmen, necessarily results in OA. Those footballers with OA usually have a history of ligament damage predating the onset of OA. However, irrespective of the cause, OA is a painful condition that can seriously impair the quality of life.

Treatments

For the majority of sufferers, arthritis is a chronic disease which passes through various stages over quite a long period; thus the management of the disease passes through different stages also. Not everyone with chronic arthritis becomes hopelessly disabled; the degree of joint damage depends on certain biological features of the disease itself, as well as appropriate treatment being given at an early stage. Most patients require a combination of different treatments, including drug therapy, sensible programmes of rest and exercise and, for some, surgery. Another treatment frequently forgotten but nonetheless extremely important for anyone with a chronic condition such as arthritis is psychological support and help. This is necessary not only for the patients, but for their families also.

Drug Therapy

There are two main forms of drug therapy aimed at controlling arthritic disease—both with anti-inflammatory action. In RA, steroids may be used as well as gold, penicillamine, chloriquine and immunosuppressants. In OA, the aspirin-like non-steroidal anti-inflammatory drugs (NSAIDS) are effective. These drugs also have analgesic actions, so they can be used for pain control in RA. Effective control of both pain and joint swelling in the early stages of RA may reduce long-term joint damage. The dosages of the drugs required for effective management of arthritis are usually quite large and can cause adverse side-effects, so patients taking them have to be monitored very carefully. Some of these hazardous side-effects, which may affect quality of life, are shown in Table 23 and are described later.

Surgery

Surgery on the elbows and hands, but particularly on large weight-bearing joints, such as the hip, can dramatically relieve pain and improve function. The techniques and prostheses used in joint arthroplasty have undergone a great deal of research and development over the past couple of decades and have produced good results. However, it is fair to say that some problems remain unresolved, with many patients requiring revision surgery within ten years. Another unforeseen problem is that joint replacement of, for example, the knee, can sometimes accelerate deterioration in the contralateral knee or ankle (Liang *et al*, 1982). Despite these difficulties, few doubt that arthroplasty is a valuable and beneficial treatment to offer patients who are suffering from intractable pain. Surgeons are currently replacing about 30,000 damaged hips a year in Great Britain, and the procedure is popular amongst the health economists who view it as a 'good buy' in terms of the cost per quality-adjusted life year (QALY). I consider the use of QALYs in more detail in Chapter 9, but Williams (1985) has estimated that a hip replacement at £750 per QALY represents good value when compared with kidney dialysis which costs £14,000 per QALY.

TABLE 23

Threats to Quality of Life in Arthritis

Physical   —Pain
           Disability
           Insomnia
           Side-effects of drug therapy
              skin rashes
              nausea and vomiting
              diarrhoea
              impotence
              Cushing's syndrome
              renal impairment
              gastrointestinal damage

Functional —Self-care
              bathing
              hair and tooth brushing, etc.
           Using the lavatory
           Getting dressed
           Turning handles, opening doors
           Preparing and eating food
           Climbing stairs

Psychosocial—Uncertainty
           Frustration
           Depression
           Loss of self-esteem
           Loss of dignity
           Dependency
           Sexual problems
           Social difficulties
           Occupational adjustments or unemployment
           Family relationship adjustments

MEASURING QUALITY OF LIFE IN ARTHRITIS

In Table 23 I have tried to group most of the threats to quality of life experienced by arthritic patients under three main headings: physical, functional and psychosocial. There have been several measures specifically designed to evaluate some aspects of the quality of life in arthritis; most of these are primarily concerned with assessment of functional status and ability to engage in the activities of daily living (see, for example, the self-assessment Arthritis Status Test shown in Table 24).

TABLE 24

A Typical Arthritis Self-Assessment Test

	Without difficulty	With difficulty	With help from another	Unable to do at all
DAILY FUNCTION				
1 Dressing: Can you get your clothes, dress yourself, shampoo your hair . . .	0	1	2	3
2 Standing up: Are you able to stand up from a chair without using your arms to push off . . .	0	1	2	3
3 Eating: Can you cut your meat and lift a cup to your mouth . . .	0	1	2	3

The main difficulty with adopting this approach is that a patient's own perceived function tends to be a relative judgement, influenced by such things as sex, age, motivation, available social supports and personal priorities and goals. It is not unusual for elderly patients, for example, to rate their functional status as good, even when they are clearly disabled.

Further questioning usually reveals that they make such judgements relative to other people of a similar age. Liang and Robb-Nicholson (1987) cite the case of an 80-year-old arthritic patient: 'His apartment was bare except for a cockpit around his couch on which he stayed 24 hours a day. He slept, drank and toileted there and his knees took the shape of his couch. He could not walk unaided.' This man, however, rated himself as having no functional limitations.

Another important point to consider when measuring quality of life following different treatments for arthritis is the time frame during which measures are made and the necessity to integrate morbidity and mortality data. In previous chapters I have drawn attention to the fact that some clinicians treating patients with highly toxic chemotherapy might well extend the *length* of life without considering the cost of that extra time in terms of lost *quality* of life if the patient suffers many months of unpleasant side-effects, such as nausea and vomiting, hair loss and mouth soreness. With RA there is a rather different problem. Treatment with steroid drugs can quickly and dramatically improve the inflamed joint, reducing the swelling and increasing mobility. Quality of life measures taken at this time may reveal an enhanced sense of well-being and much improved functional status, but long-term treatment with steroids has many associated risks which a short-term quality of life study might not pick up. Patients on long-term steroid therapy are more susceptible to infection, thus increasing their mortality, and they may experience steroid-induced fractures due to osteoporosis. The drugs may alter body shape, (the classical description is of a person with a moon-face, obesity of the trunk and wasting of the arm and leg muscles), threaten vision, cause diabetes and give rise to baldness and acne in men, and hirsutism (increased body and beard hair) in women. If the unfortunate patient is already having to cope with the disfigurement of arthritic joints, the combined assault on body-image of this, together with steroid therapy side-effects, is enormous and deeply distressing.

Another example of the importance of timing when evaluating the outcome of treatment can be seen in the impressive multicentre randomised clinical trial of auranofin in rheumatoid arthritis, reported by Bombardier and her colleagues

(1986). In this study, more than 300 patients received either auranofin or placebo. Outcome was assessed using five standard clinical measures of improvement, such as swollen joints, together with a large number of less traditional quality of life measures, including the McGill Pain Questionnaire (see Chapter 2), the Quality of Well-Being Scale (QWB) and Health Assessment (HAQ), both of which will be described later. It was only after three months that differences appeared between the two groups, with those patients given auranofin experiencing less swollen joints and a better quality of life. By six months these differences were even more apparent, with a superior quality of life reported by the auranofin group, despite the experience of certain side-effects from the drug. The quality of life tools employed in this study showed good correlation with the clinical assessments of improvement being used and provided a much broader evaluation of the efficacy of the drugs.

Tests Developed Specifically for Use in Arthritis
The American Rheumatism Association's four-point functional capacity scale, developed in 1949, has been used as the basis for most of the functional assessments in RA, in particular the well-known Arthritis Impact Measurement Scales (AIMS) of Meenan et al. (1980). The AIMS shown in Table 25 assess mobility, physical activity, dexterity, ability to perform household activities and other activities of daily living, social life, pain and finally psychological status.

The AIMS contains 48 multiple-choice questions grouped in a Guttman-type format, that is response choices form a continuum of increasing levels of intensity or severity. The scores form subscales which are added together, then averaged to find a total score. Meenan and his colleagues have researched their test well and it has been shown to have good validity and reliability.

Another test specifically designed for use in diseases such as arthritis is the Functional Status Index (FSI) of Jette (1980). The FSI measures pain, dependence and difficulty in 18 areas of daily living. There is a physician-completed version as well as a self-assessment version available (shown in Table 26).

TABLE 25

Items from the Arthritis Impact Measurement Scale (AIMS)

Social Activity

5 About how often were you on the telephone with close friends or relatives during the past month?

4 Has there been a change in the frequency or quality of your sexual relationships during the past month?

3 During the past month, about how often have you had friends or relatives to your home?

2 During the past month, about how often did you get together socially with friends or relatives?

1 During the past month, how often have you visited with friends or relatives at their homes?

Anxiety

6 During the past month, how much of the time have you felt tense or 'high strung'?

5 How much have you been bothered by nervousness, or your 'nerves' during the past month?

4 How often during the past month did you find yourself having difficulty trying to calm down?

3 How much of the time during the past month were you able to relax without difficulty?

2 How much of the time during the past month have you felt calm and peaceful?

1 How much of the time during the past month did you feel relaxed and free of tension?

TABLE 26

Functional Status Index

Composition of 5 Functional Status Categories
Derived From Factor Analysis Results

Gross Mobility	Personal Care
walking inside	washing all parts of the body
stair climbing	putting on pants
chair transfers	putting on a shirt
	buttoning a shirt

Hand Activities	Home Chores
opening containers	doing laundry
writing	reaching into low cupboards
dialing a phone	doing yardwork
	vacuuming a rug

Interpersonal Activities

driving a car
visiting family or friends
attending meetings
performing your job

The final test I want to describe (although the reader should be aware that there are many others available and in the process of being developed) is the Health Assessment Questionnaire (HAQ) of Fries *et al.* (1980). As can be seen in Table 27, this test measures the ability to perform a variety of activities of daily living and tries to assess the patient's need for assistance in satisfactorily engaging in these activities, or his or her dependence on specialised equipment. The HAQ also contains a visual analogue scale for the measurement of pain.

In an interesting paper, Liang and his colleagues (1982) compared the measurement efficiency and sensitivity of five health status instruments useful in arthritis research—the FSI, HAQ, AIMS, SIP and the Quality of Well-Being (QWB). The QWB, orginally developed by Kaplan *et al.* (1976), was administered by trained interviewers who determined mobility,

TABLE 27

Items from Health Assessment Questionnaire

	without difficulty	with difficulty	with some help from another person	unable to do?

4. WALKING
   Are you able to:

   a. walk outdoor on flat ground

5. HYGIENE
   Are you able to:

   a. wash and dry your entire body
   b. use a bathtub
   c, turn faucets on and off
   d. get on and off the toilet

6. REACH
   Are you able to:

   a. comb your hair
   b. reach and get down a 5 lb. bag
      of sugar which is above your head

7. GRIP
   Are you able to:

   a. open push-button car doors
   b. open jars which have been
      previously opened
   c. use a pen or pencil

8. ACTIVITY
   Are you able to:

   a. drive a car
      (For reasons other than arthritis)
      I do not drive
   b. run errands and shop

physical and social activity on different levels, together with an assessment of various symptoms. Using this method, they then produced a weighting of different items to compute a weighted global score. The weights assigned to levels and subgroups appear valid. Balaban *et al.* (1986) reported very similar ones in a study of patients with RA, although there do appear to be some counter-intuitive weightings, with the wearing of glasses producing a higher disability score than being in a wheelchair!

In Liang *et al.*'s comparative study, 50 patients who had undergone hip or knee replacements for either RA or OA filled in all five assessment questionnaires pre- and post-operatively. Pre-operatively the self-reported levels of both pain and physical impairment were high, with good correlations between all the quality of life instruments used. There were clear improvements in both pain and functional performance at three months post-operatively and marked differences between were observed in the ability of the tests to pick up these improvements. Particularly good at detecting the mobility improvements were the AIMS, FSI and SIP, whereas the HAQ and QWB performed half as efficiently. Only three of the instruments, the HAQ, FSI and AIMS, were compared for their efficiency in picking up the improvement in pain intensity. Of these, the FSI was superior to the others. Social function was best assessed by the FSI, although the tests all interpreted this rather differently. Interestingly, a final comparison made for the global indices of functional impairment revealed that the FSI and HAQ were less than a third as efficient as the SIP, AIMS or QWB. This finding was probably due to the emphasis given to pain as an important subscale or problem area in the latter three tests. The relevant point to consider is that different tests may well give different answers, so it is extremely important to ensure that quality of life assessment measures are truly comparable when looking at findings from different studies. This, of course, is necessary in all work for those disease states where quality of life is an outcome measure. It is possible that key areas of improvement or impairment might not be revealed if the test chosen lacked a specific subscale or enough items to determine the aspect of quality of life being considered.

The Quackery of Life in Arthritis

Any oppressive chronic disorder which cannot be cured instantly by allopathic medicine attracts the fraudulent pedlars of quack cures. I have already described some of the magical 'cures' promoted in the cancer world; the arthritis quacks are equally innovative and active, playing on the gullibility of desperate people.

Apart from losing a considerable amount of money in the search for cures which turn out to be false, some patients are coerced into abandoning orthodox treatments such as steroids or gold injections, thus compromising their health further. All the usual gimmicks are employed, especially the promotion of expensive diets, enemas and vitamin injections. Carrot and celery juice seem to be prominent, together with vitamin E in huge doses. It has been suggested that ingesting cod-liver oil will 'oil' the damaged joints, or that bee-venom desensitisation by injection 'cures' the disease. Lotions, potions, liniments and ointments for topical application, containing an extraordinary mixture of substances from lighter fuel to whisky, or banana skins, have all been promoted at different times. Acupuncture is perennially popular, but it is interesting to note that the Chinese acupuncturists have never felt it effective for the treatment of rheumatoid arthritis in China (Fries, 1979)! Organising trips for immersion in spa and mineral springs in various parts of the world is a lucrative business, improving the bank balances of the tour operators rather than the arthritis of the hopeful travellers. Wearing a copper bracelet looks attractive and is innocuous enough, but it is unlikely to be as effective as aspirin. One study found that 38 per cent of patients with RA or OA wear copper or other jewellery (Kronenfeld and Wasner, 1982). Finally, some of the wonder-drugs that are peddled under the label of natural or alternative therapy, particularly those available in clinics south of the Mexican border, usually contain cortico-steroids. Taking these in an uncontrolled manner, without professional advice and monitoring, is extremely dangerous, and people have died as a consequence.

The only enhancement to quality of life likely to be achieved by those unhappy people who solicit quack cures is a temporary improvement in symptoms. This placebo effect occurs as a result of the desire and need to feel better, in combination with any novel treatment. The false hopes perpetrated by the fraudsters hinder adjustment to chronic disease and the development of long-term coping strategies. They also undermine confidence in traditional medical practitioners who are trying hard to alleviate symptoms with scientifically tested treatments. One expert in the treatment of arthritis estimated that at least 20 per cent of his patients admitted that they had tried some form of quack medicine (Fries, 1979). This is probably an underestimate: other studies have shown that between 50 and 98 per cent of disillusioned arthritics have tried alternative methods (Walrad, 1960; Kronenfeld and Wasner, 1982). Some gained temporary relief, most were bitterly disappointed and much poorer, and some experienced the dangerous consequences of soliciting such help.

A disease characterised by remissions and exacerbations allows the spurious claims of 'cure'. It is important to note that the proof offered by the quacks for the efficacy of their methods is always anecdotal. The study by Kronenfeld and Wasner revealed that use of unorthodox therapies was virtually universal, with no significant differences between patients of different disease status, age, sex, class or educational background. The appeal of the quack cures and folk remedies highlights the hopelessness and helplessness experienced by many chronic arthritic patients. They are searching for some sense of control over their illness and clearly feel that there must be something outside orthodox treatment which will provide more relief from their suffering. To medical scientists, such behaviour might seem irrational, but the extent to which people are prepared to try anything speaks volumes for the desperation experienced by patients enduring unrelieved symptoms.

COPING WITH ARTHRITIS

The stress of coping with chronic rheumatoid arthritis appears to alter personality. A study by Crown and Crown (1973) showed that patients who had been suffering from RA for less than a year displayed a normal range of personality characteristics in comparison with the high levels of neurotic traits found in chronic sufferers. There is also some research showing that patients with more neurotic personalities seem more prone to psychiatric disturbance during the course of their illness (Gardiner, 1980). The importance of measuring personal factors and psychiatric morbidity was shown by Crown *et al*. (1975) who found that different psychological characteristics are associated with the presence or absence of rheumatoid factor in the blood serum. This finding was replicated in another study of 129 rheumatoid arthritic patients, which reported a high incidence of psychiatric morbidity. The majority of the 53 per cent of patients deemed probable psychiatric cases according to the GHQ (see Chapter 2) lacked the rheumatoid factor in their blood serum. The GHQ test scores were significantly lower for serum positive patients (Gardiner, 1980). Crown has suggested that, as the presence of rheumatoid factor in serum seems to predict a more serious form of the disease than that found in the seronegative patients, the monitoring of psychological variables at an early stage of the disease may have implications for the management of arthritis and in terms of the psychological support offered to patients.

Whilst biochemical factors may well influence mood states and ability to cope, there are clearly other features of the disease itself which affect the psychosocial well-being or quality of life of individuals with arthritis. Recently published work has identified different patterns of coping style, which have a significant influence on psychological adaptation (Newman *et al*,. 1989).

All people with arthritis have to learn to cope with pain, functional impairment, disability and sometimes deformity, together with the uncertainty as to when they will be affected, how badly, and how long the exacerbation of their illness will last. Everyone experiences areas of uncertainty in their lives, but the uncertainty endured by arthritic patients may surpass tolerable levels and demand mastery of a variety of coping strategies in order to preserve psychological well-being. In an interesting observational study of patients with RA, Carolyn Wiener (1975) identified three primary psychological and social strategies for coping with uncertainty:

a   one in which people juxtaposed their hopes for relief from symptoms and/or remission against their dread of progression and/or dependency;

b   another, where people developed strategies to try and normalise life by covering up, keeping up and pacing; and finally

c   a re-normalising strategy of periodically adjusting to reduced levels of activity.

One of Wiener's interviewees described the uncertainty of disease progression as analogous to that of owning a second-hand car. 'I think of my body like a used car, waiting for the next part to go.' Patients frequently counteract their pessimism about relapse and progression with displacement activities that may permit some sense of mastery or control over the symptoms. This is another reason why unorthodox remedies are so popular. They provide a mechanism for maintaining hope, which, because of the capricious nature of the disease, may be sustained for lengthy periods only to be dashed when the next exacerbation occurs. A loss of hope invariably means psychological dysfunction, thus maintenance of hope is a valuable coping strategy, even if it appears unrealistic. 'Even those whose deformity has made their invalidism appear to the outsider as irreversible have been socialised to the oscillations of flare-up and remission to such an extent that they continue to hope.' (Wiener, 1975).

Normalising
One means of coping is acting as though one is physically normal. Arthritic patients may do this by *covering up* the pain or trying to conceal their disability from others. By employing this strategy, the patients are not necessarily denying the reality of their disease, rather they are attempting to minimise their handicaps: '. . . it is a rejection of the social significance of the handicap and not the rejection of the handicap *per se.*' (Davis, 1973) This quotation comes from a book about living with multiple sclerosis, where similar covering up coping strategies may be employed. There are many penalties for covering up. Sometimes it fails and leads to unwanted

attention, help or advice, and if it is successful it can be immensely draining on other coping resources. Trying to disguise pain and disability is very tiring, for example, and the disease state itself does create extreme fatigue.

Successful covering up strategies may lead to optimism about *keeping up* with the normal activities of daily life, so crucial to morale and self-esteem. Wiener describes 'super normalisers' who 'engage in excessive keeping up'; a prerequisite for this is an increased pain threshold and she reports the case of a patient who had refined his keeping up and raised his pain threshold to such an extent that he walked around with a broken leg for a month, suspecting that the pain was due to arthritis. As with covering up, there are penalties for keeping up, especially increased pain and fatigue later.

There is another problem—the fact that successful covering up and keeping up might result in social acceptance and being regarded as normal, thus failing to receive appropriate sympathy, or even attracting suspicions of malingering when inactivity is forced upon the patient by an acute attack of the disease. The need to be regarded as normal, together with the need for people to be sensitive and conscious of the effort to suppress pain, is an impossible paradox which can create stress and frustration.

Pacing

One method of coping which can lead to successful covering up and keeping up is pacing, in the sense of rationing effort appropriately. Flexible pacing strategies, whereby the arthritic patient learns how to engage in activities provided that they are accompanied by a sensible appraisal of physiological status, together with rest periods, can help individuals maintain a satisfactory quality of life. This may also be linked with the periodic need to re-normalise.

Re-normalisation

This coping strategy requires patients to adjust their expectations; in particular to lower their ideas and ambitions about different physical objectives in order that achievable goals may be realised. This demands a reappraisal of some previously acquired coping strategies, especially when, for example, disease progression means that covering up is impossible. Patients who become dependent on others for help with washing, dressing, toileting or shopping, for example, and who are increasingly uncertain how long this dependency will last (indeed, they may have fears that certain functional activities will never be possible again) have to go through a successful stage of re-normalisation. The options for maintaining some sense of mastery, self-respect and self-determination in this situation may be quite limited and the threat to life's quality, moreover, may pose an intolerable burden.

CONCLUSION

Arthritis in all its forms is an oppressive chronic disorder which can severely impair the quality of life of sufferers. In this chapter I have described some of the ways in which quality of life is affected and some of the methods for measuring the impact that arthritis is having on patients' lives. Hopefully, the reader will appreciate the importance of proper measurement of quality of life variables, when evaluating the outcome of different treatments for this unpleasant chronic disease.

References

BALABAN, D.J., SAGI, P.C., GOLDFARB, N.I. and NETTLER, S. (1986). 'Weights for scoring the quality of well-being instrument among rheumatoid arthritics', in *Med. Care*, 24: 973-80.

BOMBARDIER, C., WARE, J., RUSSELL, I.J. *et al.* (1986). 'Auranofin therapy and quality of life in patients with rheumatoid arthritis: results of a multicentre trial', in *Am. J. Med.*, 81: 565-78.

CROWN, S. and CROWN, J.M. (1973). 'Personality in early rheumatoid disease', in *J. Psychosom. Res.*, 17: 189-97.

CROWN, S., CROWN, J. and FLEMING, A. (1975). 'Aspects of the psychology and epidemiology of rheumatoid disease', in *Psychol. Med.* 5: 291-9.

DAVIS, M.Z. (1973). *Living with Multiple Sclerosis: A social psychological analysis.* Springfield, Illinois: C.C. Thomas.

DOREVITCH, M.I. (1988). 'The natural history of arthritis in the elderly', in *Geriatric Medicine*, Dec: 45-8.

FRIES, J.F. (1980). *Arthritis and How to Cope With It.* London: Granada Publishing Ltd.

FRIES, J.F., SPITZ, P.W. and YOUNG, D.Y. (1982). 'The dimensions of health outcomes: the health assessment questionnaire, disability and pain scales', in *J. Rheumatology*, 9: 789–93.

GARDINER, B.M. (1980). 'Psychological aspects of rheumatoid arthritis', in *Psychol. Med.*, 10: 159–63.

HUSKISSON, E.C. (1985). *Osteoarthritis: Pathogenesis and Management.* Update Postgraduate Centre Series. London: Update Medical Education Publications.

JETTE, A.M. (1980). 'Functional status instrument: reliability of a chronic disease evaluation instrument', in *Arch. Phys. Med. Rehabil.*, 61: 395–401.

KRONENFELD, J.J. and WASNER, C. (1982). 'The use of unorthodox therapies and marginal practitioners', in *Soc. Sci. Med.*, 16(11): 1119–26.

LAWRENCE, J.S. (1977). *Rheumatism in Populations.* London: Heinemann Medical Publishing.

LIANG, M.H., CULLEN, K., LARSON, M. (1982). 'In search of a more perfect mousetrap (health status or quality of life instrument)', in *J. Rheum.*, 9(5): 775–9.

LIANG, M.H., ROBB-NICHOLSON, C. (1987). 'Health status and utility measurement viewed from the right brain: experience from the rheumatic diseases', in *J. Chron. Dis.*, 40(6): 579–83.

MEENAN, R.F., GERTMAN, P.M. and MASON, J.H. (1980). 'Measuring health status in arthritis: the Arthritis Impact Measurement Scale', in *Arthritis and Rheumatism*, 23: 146–52.

NEWMAN, S, FITZPATRICK, R. LAMB, R. and SHIPLEY, M. (1989). 'Patterns of coping in RA', in *Psychology and Health* (in press).

WALRAD, R. (1960). *The misrepresentation of arthritis drugs and devices in the U.S.* Arthritis and Rheumatism Foundation.

WIENER, C. (1975). 'The burden of rheumatoid arthritis: tolerating the uncertainty', in *Soc. Sci. Med.*, 9: 97–104.

WILLIAMS, A. (1985). 'Economics of coronary artery bypass grafting', in *BMJ*, 291: 326–9.

7 THE QUALITY OF LIFE IN THE ELDERLY

Sans teeth, sans eyes, sans taste, sans everything.
As You Like It, Act II, Sc. 2

Shakespeare painted a rather bleak picture of what it means to grow old in Jaques' 'Seven Ages of Man' speech. Worse still, this description is confined only to the physical deterioration experienced. For many elderly people he might also have added: sans self-esteem, personal efficacy, love, companionship and social support. All but the most fiercely independent amongst us need to feel, according to Cobb (1976), loved and cared for; esteemed and valued; and a sense of belonging 'to a network of communication and mutual obligation'. Without these supports many old people experience a psychological impotence leading to a state of helpless hopelessness, graphically described as a 'giving-up given-up' syndrome by Engel (1968).

Such a psychologically compromised state may either lead to the development of disease through a complex effect on neuroimmunologic pathways, or precipitate physical deterioration and disease through self-neglect. The elderly giving-up given-up person has an increased need for social supports to provide help, love, reassurance and enhancement of self-respect, but perversely he or she is often functioning in an environment devoid of the social relationships likely to provide these things. There are, of course, many age-related life-events which provoke these psycho-social problems, but the three major concomitants of old age that profoundly affect the quality of life are: 1) physical and mental deterioration; 2) retirement; and 3) bereavement. I shall discuss quality of life in all three areas later on in this chapter, but first I shall describe some of the most commonly used assessment measures employed to determine aspects of quality of life in elderly people.

TABLE 28

CLIFTON ASSESSMENT PROCEDURES FOR THE ELDERLY (CAPE)
Survey Version

Name:
Current address/placement:
Date of birth: Age:
Information/Orientation

Name:	Hospital/Address	Colour of Flag:
Age:	City:	Day:
D.O.B.	P.M:	Month:
Ward/Place	U.S. President	Year:

Physical disability

1/0 Score . . .

1. When bathing or dressing, he/she requires:
   —no assistance   0
   —some assistance   1
   —maximum assistance   2

2. With regard to walking, he/she:
   —shows no signs of weakness   0
   —walks slowly without aid, or uses a stick   1
   —is unable to walk, or if able to walk
    needs frame, crutches or someone by
    his/her side   2

3. He/she is incontinent of urine and/or faeces (day or night):
   —never   0
   —sometimes (once or twice per week)   1
   —frequently (3 times per week or more)   2

4. He/she is in bed during the day (bed does not include couch, settee, etc)
   —never   0
   —sometimes   1
   —almost always   2

5. He/she is confused (unable to find way around, loses possessions, etc):
   —almost never confused   0
   —sometimes confused   1
   —almost always confused   2

6. When left to his/her own devices, his/her appearance (clothes and/or hair) is:
   —almost never disorderly   0
   —sometimes disorderly   1
   —almost always disorderly   2

Pd Score

Measuring Disability in the Elderly

Probably the most well-known measures of behavioural and cognitive functioning in the elderly are the Clifton Assessment Procedures for the Elderly (CAPE), developed by Pattie and Gilleard (1979). The CAPE has two parts: a Cognitive Assessment Scale (CAS) and a Behaviour Rating Scale (BRS). These can be used separately or together, depending on the requirements of the clinician or researcher. For survey work Pattie (1981) has published a shortened assessment called the CAPE Survey Version, shown in Table 28. The CAS element contains three subscales: a 12-item assessment of information and orientation (e.g. What is your name? Who is the current prime minister?); a mental ability test assessing reading and writing, the ability to recite the alphabet and to count; and finally a psychomotor test based on the Gibson Spiral Maze (Gibson, 1977).

The BRS element comprises 18 items divided into four subscales of physical disability (pd), apathy (ap), communication difficulties (cd) and social disturbance (sd). Items are rated on a three-point scale by the primary care-giver (usually a relative). The scores on each subscale can be summed to give a total maximum possible score of 36. The authors offer a grading system from A-E, derived from the numerical scores. This grading scheme has been used to determine where patients should be placed for appropriate care, although the authors never intended that it should be used in this way. The shortened survey version of the CAPE is extremely useful for large population studies or when several other tests and measures are being employed. It is easy to understand, quick to complete and can be administered by people after very little training.

Apart from chronic disability, old age frequently heralds chronic depressive illness; together these problems can severely impair quality of life. One measure which has been used to examine throughly the relationship between disability and depression in elderly people is the Comprehensive Assessment and Referral Evaluation (CARE) of Gurland *et al.* (1977). The CARE is a semi-structured questionnaire administered by trained interviewers. It probes many areas of physical, psychological and social functioning, together with assessment of functional status and utilisation of medical and social

TABLE 29

Assessment areas in the CARE

Area	Typical Items
Physical	Evidence of cancer Heart disease Arthritis Bowel problems Hearing, visual and dental problems Self-rating of health
Psychological	Memory Depressed mood Anxiety Sleep disorders Delusions/hallucinations
Social Problems	Isolation Family relationships Perception of 'being a burden' Retirement adjustment Finances
Habits	Eating Smoking Drugs/alcohol abuse
Functional Status	Communication Mobility Activities of daily living
Utilisation of Services	Medical Social services Informal/voluntary help

services (see Table 29). It is therefore an extremely comprehensive quality of life schedule. The activity limitation
subscale alone has 39 items ranging from self-care tasks to
ability to carry out household chores.

In a mammoth collaborative project done by the Columbia
University Center for Geriatrics in the United States and the
Institute of Psychiatry in London, the CARE was used to

study depression and disability of patients over 65 years old (Gurland *et al.*, 1983). I cannot do justice to the volumes of impressive and detailed analyses carried out in this project, but I shall summarise some of their findings.

Gurland *et al.* reported that 13 per cent of the elderly living in the community were 'pervasively depressed', in other words suffering from depressive symptoms that warranted clinical intervention. At least 30 per cent were dependent on someone else for personal assistance to enable them to continue living in the community, another third were classified as having minor PTD (personal time dependency), with the remainder requiring almost constant personal assistance as they were completely housebound and disabled. There were more personal time-dependent elderly amongst widowed females, particularly in the oldest age groups. A high correlation was found between PTD and evidence of pervasive depression; furthermore there was a statistically significant correlation between severity of this dependency and severity of depression. If the primary care-giver was another elderly person, then this companion was at high risk of being depressed also.

Gurland *et al.* concluded that the main cause of chronic depression amongst elderly people was chronic disability and loss of independence, although other factors such as social isolation, an unsatisfactory retirement, unpleasant environment, and money worries also played a role. Importantly, they stressed that good service support from the care-giving agencies ameliorated both disability and depression, hence the necessity to maintain adequate resources for active therapeutic work amongst the elderly. On the positive side, the study showed that the proportion of elderly people who are *not* depressed despite their disabilities increases with age. These old-old seem to be more accepting and to have adjusted to their disability. It highlights the need to be optimistic and to set positive goals for therapeutic interventions and rehabilitation of elderly people who are both depressed and disabled.

Many of the quality of life instruments described in Chapter 2 have been used in elderly populations. It is always important to consider that different age groups might have rather different expectations and desires, so threshold scores for tests should, if possible, have different age-related norms.

Similarly, there are sex differences in the perception of health status amongst the elderly. Fillenbaum (1976) gave men and women over the age of 65 years, both in the community and in institutional care, a self-assessment questionaire, the Older American's Resources and Services Questionnaire (OARS). The OARS, developed by Pfeiffer (1975), measures functioning in five domains: social, economic, mental health, physical health and activities of daily living. Self-ratings of health were checked with objective assessments of health status and revealed that although women had objectively poorer health than men, women appear able to tolerate more health difficulties. Not only do women experience more health problems, but often these problems are more severe than those suffered by men (Verbrugge, 1976). Nevertheless, males with less disability and fewer illnesses rate themselves as experiencing poorer health. A later study of self-ratings of health in more than 3,000 elderly people reported similar findings and emphasised that self-assessments of health were valid, economical means of gathering information, provided that both age and sex of the respondents are controlled for (Ferraro, 1980).

One further point about measuring quality of life in the elderly concerns the prevalence of dementia. Seriously demented or cognitively impaired people cannot fill in self-assessment questionnaires or co-operate with interviews. They may require rather specialised neuropsychological assessments. Interested readers may find helpful two recently published books by Wattis and Hindmarch (1988) and Pitt (1987). I shall describe only one well-researched instrument, originally named the Kendrick Battery for the Detection of Dementia in the Elderly (KBDDE), developed by Gibson and Kendrick (1979), but now referred to as Kendrick Cognitive Tests for the Elderly (KCTE). In fact, the KCTE is really two tests: an object learning and a digit copying test. It has been shown to have extremely good reliability and validity and appears to differentiate well between the 'normal' elderly and those showing signs of dementia. It seems a useful test for both diagnosis and typing of different dementias and can be used as a screening instrument in large populations (Kendrick, 1985).

Of course, determining the cognitive status of an individual is not the same thing as measuring quality of life. I have described the KCTE here because dementia affects quality of life, not only of the sufferer, but of his or her carers, in a profound and often devastating manner, as we shall see later on in this chapter.

PHYSICAL DEGENERATION AND DISEASES OF OLD AGE

Good health probably contributes more to the overall quality of an individual's life than anything else. Failing health and infirmity are the main worries people express about growing old. The ageing process produces quite obvious external bodily changes, such as hair loss and wrinkling of the skin, and there are observable functional changes such as failing eyesight, hearing and agility, all of which affect the quality of life. An acquaintance trying to describe being old to my young son, asked him to imagine having his glasses smeared with vaseline, cotton wool stuck in his ears and walking around with stones in his shoes!

Old age does not necessarily mean decrepit senility, however, and the majority (75 per cent) of people over 65 in this country, remain physically quite fit and alert. Comfort (1977) has argued that much of the stereotypical infirmity associated with old age is culturally rather than biologically determined. This is an important point, as one frequently hears people preface statements about the elderly with comments such as, 'Of course, at his age you wouldn't expect him to be able to . . .' or, 'When you get to that age you shouldn't . . .' Thus a self-fulfilling prophecy occurs with, for example, elderly people slowing down because they *expect* to be slowed down. Likewise, they might cease sexual activity because they are culturally conditioned to myths that sexual desire is inappropriate in old age rather than actually experiencing a loss of desire. Evidence for this can be seen in a questionnaire study done by Hendricks and Hendricks (1978). They asked people aged between 60 and 93 years about their sexual activity. Results revealed little decline in their respondents' previous, more youthful, sexual activity and interest up to the age of 75 years. Even at 75 years 25 per cent of the sample were still sexually active.

Whilst there is an exaggerated belief that old age inevitably means ill-health, one cannot ignore the fact that certain sorts of diseases and degenerative changes affect predominantly the elderly. Most of the common cancers and cardiovascular disorders are age-related, as are certain orthopaedic/rheumatic complaints and cerebral changes. Although physical evidence of many of these diseases can be detected in the elderly, they do not always result in disabling functional impairments. Not everyone with mild atheroma has obvious coronary heart disease, for example. On the other hand, some old people may suffer multiple pathologies severely impairing their quality of life.

When measuring the quality of any individual's life, it is of course important to ascertain just how much interference a particular disease or symptom is exerting on everyday aims and tasks. It is sometimes rather difficult to quantify the relative disadvantage different disorders exert on everyday functioning. For example, angina or breathlessness when walking upstairs might be seen as a major disruption to the life of an elderly man who previously enjoyed activities such as walking, cycling or swimming, but this might seem a minimal problem in comparison with the difficulty of another person unable to bend and cut his own toenails, or with the problems of someone unable to read due to cataracts or diabetic retinopathy. The mere fact that one disorder is significantly more life-threatening than another might have little to do with how much disruption to daily activities and enjoyment of life the symptoms of disease produce.

Just as old age is taken by many to be synonymous with ill-health, it is also viewed as a period of inevitable gloom, despondency and depression. Elaine Murphy (1986), in her excellent book *Affective Disorders in the Elderly* cites this quotation from Robert Burton's *Anatomy of Melancholy* (1652):

Old age, which being cold and dry and of the same quality as melancholy is, must needs cause it. Melancholy . . . is a necessary and inseparable accident of all old and decrepit persons. After 70 years, all is trouble and sorrow . . .

This natural infirmity is most eminent in old women and such as are poor, solitary, live in base esteem and beggary.

There is plenty of evidence to show, however, that provided elderly people are not severely disabled and/or if they have good social and practical support available to them, depression is not inevitable. Unfortunately, those elderly people who do suffer from depressive illness are most unlikely to be recognised as depressed, let alone referred on for help to a psychiatrist (Shepherd, 1980). This is partially due to the fact that elderly patients do not report their depression to doctors. MacDonald (1985) showed that GPs tend to be rather apathetic about active psychiatric help for their patients. Although the GPs in this study recognised those elderly patients who were depressed (in fact they often over-diagnosed depression), there was a notable reluctance to refer on for specialist care or to prescribe anti-depressants.

Proper diagnosis and treatment of depression in the elderly is important for several reasons, not the least of which is the fact that depression can be the presenting sign of a wide variety of physical illnesses. Myxoedema, pernicious anaemia, cancer and neurosyphilis, for example, can all present with depression. Perversely, the drugs used to treat some physical illnesses can also cause depression, particularly the anti-hypertensive drugs such as reserpine, methyldopa and propanolol. Richer *et al.* (1983) showed that 24 per cent of the elderly patients studied in one general practice were taking a drug likely to *cause* depression.

As I have already mentioned, the CARE study showed a significant correlation between depression and disability. Depressed elderly patients are less likely to cope with physical disability; indeed, the self-neglect and loss of self-esteem, insomnia and loss of appetite all precipitate physical deterioration and lead to the need for institutional care. Apart from the obvious humanitarian need to investigate, diagnose and *treat* depression in the elderly, it may well be cost effective if the patient can then remain in the community.

The health-related quality of life experienced by the elderly is influenced to a major extent by the amount of resources made available for their care. We have an increasingly elderly population in this country. A recent report from the Royal College of Physicians estimated that more than one million people in the United Kingdom will be aged 85 years or over by the end of this century.

As there is currently such poor funding and poor co-ordination between the Departments of Health and Social Security and local authorities for the provision of adequate care facilities for our elderly, the future gives cause for extreme concern. The private sector is not attracted to the development of care services which elderly people could afford, and geriatrics is not a medical speciality attractive to many doctors and nurses. Hence we have inadequate financial provision for services, a dearth of care facilities, and an acute manpower shortage; the report from the Royal College of Physicians (1989) referred to above, revealed, for example, that at the end of 1986 over 30 per cent of the elderly in the United Kingdom had no psycho-geriatric service at all. Not surprisingly, nursing care often falls on the long-suffering (and largely unsupported) relatives and friends of elderly people. This can prove an intolerable burden, as such care can be intensely wearing, especially if the elderly person is suffering from dementia. It has been estimated that approximately one in every 25 people over the age of 65 years, and one in every five over the age of 80, show clinical evidence of dementia, in particular Alzheimer's Disease. Studies using the CAPE information/orientation subscale have reported that between two and four per cent of over-65-year-olds have dementia (Pattie, 1988).

Alzheimer's Disease

Alzheimer's Disease is the most common of all the dementias, affecting as many as 500,000 people in the United Kingdom (Roth and Iverson, 1986). Due to the predicted increase in the elderly population by the turn of the century, and the realisation that we fail to cope adequately with the elderly Alzheimer's patients currently living in this country, there has been renewed interest in the cause of the disease and possible means of preventing or treating it. One thing is quite clear: we are most unlikely to have anything like the necessary resources to look after all the demented elderly people requiring specialist institutions. Primary care will almost certainly remain the responsibility of relatives.

There have been many debates in the literature over the past 30 years concerning the most appropriate diagnostic criteria for Alzeimer's Disease. Current criteria require neuropathological as well as clinical signs and symptoms. At post-mortem there are characteristic senile plaques and neurofibrillary tangles in the brains of sufferers. Patients also seem to have deficiencies of important neurotransmitter substances, such as dopamine, noradrenaline and serotonin.

As far as clinical features are concerned, there appear to be three stages in the development of the disease. The initial stage is marked by a sudden and obvious memory impairment, and patients usually still have some insight and awareness of their difficulties. This memory deficit is accompanied by problems with naming quite common items, and affected individuals often show signs of a fixed, forward-staring gaze. In the second stage of the disease, there is evidence of progressive dementia; memory becomes much more disturbed, with a large number of neuropsychological deficits—disorientation, agraphia, alexia, aphasia, perseveration, apraxia, and dysarthria, to name but a few. Patients often have a disturbed gait and muscle tone and usually become incontinent. In the final stage of this awful disease, patients are frequently mute, stuporous and in a vegetative state; they often have pressure sores and can end up severely emaciated. Death is usually due to secondary infections, such as pneumonia—'the old man's friend' (Gruenberg, 1977).

As patients may suffer from other physical problems, and secondary psychiatric disorders, as well as those mentioned above, even the most experienced clinician may have difficulty in determining the relative contribution that each component may be exerting on the overall disability of the unfortunate patient, and his or her quality of life.

One thing is certain, the burden of caring for a person with Alzheimer's Disease is wearing and exasperating to the extent that quality of life for the primary care-giver is severely impaired. Whether or not care is provided out of love for, or duty towards the patient, many relatives find themselves close to breaking point and the presence of the patient can provoke the destruction of marital and family relationships.

In the early stages of the illness, most relatives notice a change in mood state. Patients may become depressed or emotionally rather flat; they also show signs of agitation and anxiety, especially when the amnesia deepens. Relatives and other care-givers can be driven to the limits of their patience by the repeated questioning and demands for reassurance. Constant repetition of questions about the time or what day it is, or who the person at the door was, can be intensely irritating. As the disease progresses, patients may forget how to dress: they may use the wrong armhole in clothes, for example, or become unable to tie up shoelaces. They sometimes fail to recognise the faces of other family members and even have problems with their own reflection in a mirror. Often they become extremely disorientated and insist on following their spouses around the house. If left alone, they may wander out of the house and get completely lost. Needless to say, this causes profound confusion and bewilderment and some care-givers become socially isolated as they dare not leave their relatives alone. For some relatives it becomes increasingly difficult to maintain love and respect for the agitated, anxious, densely amnesic patient, who bears little resemblance to the person they once knew.

Apart from the emotional trauma, there are many other problems that carers must face. There is the physical exhaustion provoked by the heavy nursing care which some patients require, together with the difficulty of constant broken nights, for sufferers who are disorientated often wake and wander around at night. Patients with advanced disease may be incontinent, which may pose a further source of considerable stress on the carer, especially if he or she has no laundry service provided by the local authority.

Frequently, women are emotionally blackmailed into caring for an elderly parent or parent-in-law. This can cause marital disharmony and acute difficulties for grandchildren, who may be too embarrassed by their demented grandparent's behaviour to invite friends home. In view of the increasing numbers of elderly patients who will have to be cared for in the community, there is an urgent need to start planning adequate support services to assist relatives in coping with the task. The quality of life of the whole family can be threatened by the presence of a patient with Alzheimer's Disease.

THE EFFECTS OF RETIREMENT ON QUALITY OF LIFE

In 1981, the Census shows that there were 7,985,102 elderly (that is of pensionable age—65+) living in Great Britain. Table 30 shows a more detailed breakdown of that figure by age and sex.

TABLE 30

People of pensionable age living in Great Britain (1981)

Age (in years)	65-74	75-84	85-94	94+
Total No.	4,932,307	2,500,408	521,786	30,601
% men	43.8	34.6	23.8	17.9
% women	56.2	65.4	76.2	82.1

One interesting point to ponder is that fewer men than women even reach retirement age and of those who do, most die sooner than women. Furthermore, almost three-quarters of elderly men are married, whereas nearly two thirds of elderly women are either single or widowed. There are variations in retirement age depending on the rules of different employing organisations and professions, but the state pension only becomes payable (with the exception of those forced into early retirement by ill health) at 65 years of age for men and 60 for women, although recent changes mean that many women will now have the option to continue working until 65 years.

Retirement from full-time paid employment is a major life event, producing radical changes in virtually all aspects of an individual's life. The gains from relinquishing the burdensome toil of everyday labour are often offset by the losses in income, social contact and certain other important 'role losses'. Although many people are well-prepared for retirement and have made plans to move house, take up some voluntary employment or devote more time to a pursuit or hobby which they were unable to follow while working, others find that they have lost a major reference group which used to provide them with a sense of identity and social contact. For those somewhat 'traditional' family structures where the woman is the childcarer and homemaker and the man seen as the breadwinner, retirement can produce considerable marital disharmony and resentment. The husband will often attempt to establish routines within the home which will fulfil the needs which employment used to satisfy, especially those of feeling useful and competent. Not surprisingly, many women resent surrendering their role of household organiser and conflict can develop.

Other stresses result from the sudden loss of income accompanying retirement. Not all elderly people have handsome golden handshakes and good retirement pensions from their erstwhile employers. Tables 31a and 31b reveal the stark reality of financial hardship endured by many old people in this country, who have little other than the basic state pension to live on. When essentials such as food, housing and heating are paid for, over 40 per cent of elderly households have little to spare for household repairs or big power bills if there has been a particularly severe winter.

TABLE 31a

Average weekly income (in pounds)	Elderly household (containing average 1.7 people)	Non-elderly (containing average 3.1 people)
Less than 55	40.4%	5.7%
Over 55, less than 120	41.1%	20.1%
Over 120, less than 200	11.9%	33.8%
Over 200	6.6%	40.4%

Apart from the obvious threats to health if income is insufficient for adequate food, clothing, heating and housing, a low fixed income considerably restricts the ability to participate in leisure activities. Thus the improved opportunities for the newly-retired to engage in all kinds of pursuits denied many people during their working lives, due to insufficient time or competing demands when raising a family, are not realised. Some close-knit families are able to provide their retired parents with financial support, and grandchildren may also be a source of recreational activity. Furthermore, the retired person can be immensely helpful and find a new sense of

TABLE 31b

How This Money is Spent

Item	Elderly outgoings	Non-elderly outgoings
Food	17.03	30.69
Housing	15.56	21.20
Services	8.47	15.69
Transport	7.27	22.61
Fuel for heating, lighting, etc.	6.25	7.88
'Other goods', cleaning materials, etc.	4.73	11.06
Clothing	3.99	11.02
Furniture, household appliances	3.44	11.43
Alcohol	2.68	7.21
Tobacco	1.80	4.40
Miscellaneous	.21	.71
	71.43	143.90

(All figures based on 1981 census data)

purpose or role in providing child-care or baby-sitting. All these things, however, depend also on the geographic proximity of relatives. and the quality of the relationship between family members prior to retirement.

THE EFFECT OF BEREAVEMENT ON QUALITY OF LIFE

The quality of elderly people's lives is determined to a degree by their ability to adjust to loss. We have looked at the losses sustained on retirement in terms of status, income and social contact, and the loss of the physical and cognitive functioning due to age-related disease or degeneration, but the next major loss to cope with in old age is often the death of life-long partners and friends. Despite the inevitability of death as we age, bereavement is nonetheless a severely distressing and painful experience and some people never quite come to terms with their grief. A sad example of this can be seen in the diaries of Dora Carrington, who committed suicide after the death of her life-long companion, Lytton Strachey:

> They say one must keep your standards and your values of life alive. But how can I when I only kept them for you. I loved life just because you made it so perfect . . . It is impossible to think that I shall never sit with you again and hear your laugh. That every day for the rest of my life you will be away.

Some researchers, for example Neugarten (1979), have suggested that the elderly are extremely resilient to stressful life events, such as bereavement, provided that these changes occur at the 'right' time in the life-cycle. This argument stems from a notion that if events are 'on cue', for example an elderly spouse dying after a long illness, then the anticipation of such a death makes it easier to work through and adapt to the necessary changes. Old people are much more distressed by 'unfair', unexpected losses, such as the death of a middle-aged child, or a grandchild. It is true, however, that not everyone shares these ideas about the effect that bereavement has on elderly people.

Bereavement has been associated with a greater illness and mortality risk, especially for men with few social contacts (Rowland, 1977). One of the foremost researchers in this field is Colin Murray Parkes. With his colleagues, in 1969 he studied a sample of nearly 4,500 widowers aged 55 years or more. During the first six months of bereavement 213 of them died, which represented a 40 per cent increase over the expected death rate for this age group. Furthermore, the incidence of illness in the bereaved group was a staggering 67 per cent higher than for the general population (Parkes *et al.*, 1969).

Most elderly men are, however, still married (approximately three out of every four). In contrast, almost two thirds of the elderly female population are either widowed, divorced or never married. With increasing age the likelihood of a woman being alone due to the earlier death of a husband or because she never married, increases dramatically. According to figures based on the 1981 census, over 90 per cent of women aged 85-89 years are either single or widowed. Only 34 per cent over the age of 65 share their old age with a husband. Few get the opportunity to test the truth of Robert Browning's lines from the poem *Rabbi ben Ezra*: 'Grow old along with me! The best is yet to be.'

Many more experience the fear and loneliness captured in these lines written by an elderly woman named Kate who was assumed by her nurses to be senile, until they cleared out her bedside locker after her death and found a moving poem about her life and feelings on growing old: 'Dark days are upon me, my husband is dead, I look at the future, I shudder with dread.'

The grief response following bereavement appears to have certain universal characteristics, in particular the widowed person's preoccupation with the deceased partner, and pining. Researchers such as Parkes (1972) have identified a series of changes, or progressive phases, suggesting that grief is an active, evolving process, not simply a painful emotional experience which diminishes in intensity with time. This grieving process usually takes several months, reaching a peak of intensity at around six months, but as many as two thirds of widows may still be actively grieving a year or more after bereavement. The phases described by Parkes occurred in approximately 70 per cent of his subjects studied, in varying intensities. Thus they provide a useful guide to what are 'normal' reactions following death of a loved one, and what is likely to be indicative of psychiatric morbidity needing intervention.

In the first phase, most bereaved people experience a period of *numbness*. They describe feeling shocked or stunned (in a similar manner to the initial reactions of a patient on hearing that he or she has cancer). This emotional blunting and numbness can temporarily relieve the intense pain of bereavement. The second phase has been described as *separation anxiety*, with the bereaved person preoccupied with thoughts about her dead partner and an intense period of pining. Some people embark upon a phase of active, unconscious searching for the lost person. This is often followed by feelings of anger and guilt. As the yearning for the lost person subsides and the anger diminishes, many people lapse into a phase of apathy and depression. Unless they can emerge from this stage, make a new role and adapt to a new way of living, they may be more vulnerable to a wide variety of other physical diseases.

Apart from having to restructure their life without a partner and coping with the emotional and practical difficulties this entails, many widows and widowers are relatively impoverished. Table 31a, which is based on the 1981 census data, showed that 40.4 per cent of 'elderly households' (defined as one in which the head of the house was aged 65 years plus) had a weekly income of under £55. Interestingly enough, exactly the same percentage of 'non-elderly' households (40.4 per cent) had a weekly income of £200 or more. It should be noted when examining these figures that the average industrial wage in 1981 was £116.80 per week. Evidence given by Layard to the Royal Commission on the Distribution of Income and Wealth revealed that the greatest incidence of poverty was amongst widowed and single women aged 60 and above.

The consequences of physical deterioration, retirement and bereavement are often inadequate income, inappropriate housing, loneliness and social isolation. A survey carried out amongst elderly people by Age Concern in 1974 asked them to name the two worst problems which they had to face in daily life: loneliness was mentioned by 83 per cent; money by 43 per cent; poor health by 33 per cent; lack of help by 26 per cent; and bad housing by 13 per cent. Many of these difficulties could be ameliorated if governments were truly committed to the allocation of appropriate funds for our social and health services, and to community care. A rampant 'ageism' exists in our culture, with elderly people being considered as a 'problem' in much the same way as other victimised ethnic minority groups, or those with little power such as the handicapped or mentally ill. The transition from a valued, respected individual used to coping with choices and assuming some authority in various work, domestic and community situations, to a position of disregard, lacking power and influence, can be emotionally and physically devastating. Not surprisingly, most studies show that if elderly people are allowed to remain active, independent members of their family, or if they live in an enlightened nursing home that encourages self-reliance, than they experience far fewer psychological problems and are able to face the burdens imposed by other age-related life-crises more effectively (Hall, 1976).

Quality of life amongst the institutionalised elderly

At the time of the 1981 census, only three per cent of elderly people were usually resident in institutions such as homes, hospital, hostels and hotels. The last available figures (1984) showed that there were approximately 280,000 places for the elderly in England in various institutions (Larder, 1986). At that time, approximately two fifths of these places were in private nursing and rest homes. Provision of beds by the local authorities had changed little over the period between 1982 and 1984, and the number of geriatric beds within the NHS had declined. These factors, together with changes to the supplementary benefits rules which permit residents to be supported by social security payments in the private sector, have led to a dramatic increase in the number of private residential homes. Although these are regulated by local authorities, there is deep concern that such places have extremely variable standards of care, particularly as the sum payable by the Social Security has been frozen for the last four years and is now notably inadequate. This is not to say that quality of care is necessarily any better in any of the local authority or NHS institutions. The controversial 1986 annual report of the Health Advisory Service, which looked at standards of care in geriatric hospitals in England and Wales, stated that most operated in a manner which denied 'privacy, self-determination, choice, rehabilitation, psychological support and homely environments'. Furthermore, the treatment offered by some was of 'devastatingly low quality'. The thoughtful review by Day and Klein (1987) suggested that as far as the maintenance of high standards of care was concerned, the problems were 'common to all forms of institutional care for the elderly, whether public or private, whether provided by the NHS or the local authorities'. In their article Day and Klein point out the lack of any concrete definitions of standards of care which could mean a satisfactory quality of life for those unfortunate enough to depend on a residential home for the rest of their lives. They highlight the many difficulties:

> Looking after frail, confused and incontinent old people is extraordinarily demanding, both physically and emotionally, and may at times become unbearably so.

Moreover, it is a function which often tends to be left for much of the day and most of the night to the least trained, least skilled and least well-paid members of staff: aides, auxiliaries and domestics.

Incontinence in the elderly, like depression, can often be corrected after proper analysis by an expert. All too often the cost of the specialist nurse is not found, while huge sums are spent on continuing incontinence care. It has been suggested that up to half of all elderly incontinent people could have their problem corrected or much improved.

It seems a sorry reflection of public attitudes that those most dependent on good quality care are least likely to get it. The Social Services Inspectorate, reporting on residential care for the elderly in Southwark, noted that:

Life for the residents of the elderly people's homes was satisfactory, even interesting, for those who were mobile, articulate and independent. For disabled, frail or confused residents, however, the homes were failing to provide basic care and support to a satisfactory standard.

Moos *et al.* (1979, 1983) have developed a comprehensive assessment procedure for determining those aspects of an institutional environment which either enhance or diminish the quality of life of elderly people. His Multiphasic Environmental Assessment Procedure (MEAP) contains five standardised scales which evaluate such things as the building, the staff and their attitudes to care, safety features, and aids and equipment. Other researchers, such as Wells and Singer (1988), have shown the usefulness of the MEAP in helping staff to improve the quality of life in long-term care institutions. With good will, a little more imagination and committed funding, there is no reason why the quality of life for so many elderly people in this country has to remain so bleak.

CONCLUSION
Many other cultures, especially those of the Third World, do not require research theses to demonstrate the benefits for the elderly when they are held in esteem and revered for their sagacity, instead of being derided or dismissed for their frailties.

It is often our own attitudes towards the elderly which promote their declining quality of life, rather than intrinsic difficulties which they might have in coping with the inevitable consequences of ageing. With just a small amount of extra practical help, together with a more positive attitude towards correcting the physical health of elderly people, many more could enjoy an independent, satisfying finale to their lives. In the words of Elaine Murphy again:

> Small gains in physical status may alter the demoralised belief of hopelessness in the face of physical adversity and, to this end, the doctor might call upon the help of a physiotherapist or occupational therapist. Most crucial is the need to avoid colluding with the patient that decay and pain are part of old age.

Examination of the statistics shows the increase in the numbers of elderly in this country, and the obvious deficiency in the financial resources made available for providing such things as basic health care, housing and social security benefits. There is little reason for optimism about the likely quality of life most old people will experience by the end of this century.

References

BURTON, R. (1652). *Anatomy of Melancholy*, 13th ed 1827. London: Longman, Rees, Orme & Co.

COBB, S. (1976). 'Social support as a moderator of life stress', in *Psychometric Medicine*, 38: 300–14.

COMFORT, A. (1977). *A Good Age.* London: Mitchell Beazley Publishers Ltd.

DAY, P. and KLEIN, R. (1987). 'Quality of institutional care and the elderly: policy issues and options', in *BMJ*, Feb; 294: 384–7.

ENGEL, G.L. (1968). 'A life setting conducive to illness: The giving-up-given-up complex', in *Bulletin of the Menniger Clinic*, 32: 355–65.

FERRARO, K.F. (1980). 'Self-ratings of health among the old and old-old', in *J. Health and Soc. Behaviour*, 21: 377–83.

FILLENBAUM, G.G. (1976). 'Social context and self-assessments of health among the elderly', in *J. of Health and Soc. Behaviour*, 20: 45–51.

GIBSON, H.B. (1977). *Manual of the Gibson Spiral Maze*, 2nd ed. London: Hodder & Stoughton.

GIBSON, A.J. and KENDRICK, D.C. (1979). *The Kendrick Battery for the Detection of Dementia in the Elderly*. Windsor: NFER-Nelson.

GRUENBERG, E.M. (1977). 'The failures of success', in *Milbank Memorial Fund Quarterly: Health and Society*, 55(1): 3–24.

GURLAND, B.J., KURIANSKY, J.B., SHARPE, L. *et al.* (1977). 'The comprehensive assessment and referral evaluation (CARE)—rationale, development and reliability', in *Int. J. of Ageing and Human Dev.* 8: 9–42.

GURLAND, B.J., COPELAND, J.R.M., KELLEHER, M. *et al.* (1983). *The mind and mood of ageing: the mental health problems of the community elderly in New York and London*. New York: Haworth Press.

HALL, C.M. (1976). 'Ageing and family processes', in *J. of Family Counselling*, 4: 28–42.

HENDRICKS, J. and HENDRICKS, C. (1978). 'Sexuality in later life', in Carver, V. and Liddiard, P. (Eds). *An Ageing Population*. Hodder & Stoughton and Open University Press, pp. 64–71.

KENDRICK, D.C. (1985). *The Kendrick Cognitive Tests for the Elderly*. Windsor: NFER-Nelson.

KING'S FUND (1985). *Living well into old age. Applying the principles of good practice to services for elderly people with severe mental difficulties*. London: King Edward's Hospital Fund for London.

LARDER, D., DAY, P. and KLEIN, R. (1986). 'Institutional care for the elderly: the geographical distribution of the public/private mix in England', in *Bath social policy paper* No. 10. Bath: Centre for the Analysis of Social Policy.

MACDONALD, A.J.D. (1985). 'The prevalence and recognition of depressive states in elderly general practice surgery attenders'. Cited by Mann, A. and Graham, N. in Murphy, E. (Ed), *Affective Disorders in the Elderly*. Edinburgh: Churchill Livingstone, p. 152.

MOOS, R.H., GAUVAIN, M., LEMKE, S. *et al.* (1979). 'Assessing the social environments of sheltered care settings', in *The Gerontologist*, 19: 76–82.

Moos, R.H., Lemke, S. and Clayton, J. (1983). 'Comprehensive assessment of residential programs: A means of evaluation and change', in *Interdis Topics in Gerontology*, 17: 69–83.

Murphy, E. (1986). *Affective Disorders in the Elderly.* Edinburgh: Churchill Livingstone.

Neugarten, B. (1979). 'Time, age and the life cycle', in *Am. J. Psychiatry*, 136: 887–94.

Parkes, C.M. (1972). *Bereavement: studies of grief in adult life.* New York: International Universities Press.

Parkes, C.M., Benjamin, B. and Fitzgerald, R.G. (1969). 'Broken heart: a statistical study of increased mortality among widowers', in *BMJ*, 1: 740.

Pattie, A.H. and Gilleard, C.J. (1979). *Manual of the Clifton Assessment Procedures for the Elderly (CAPE).* London: Hodder & Stoughton.

Pattie, A.H. (1988). 'Measuring levels of disability—the Clifton Assessment Procedures for the Elderly', in Wattis, J.P. and Hindmarch, I. (Eds). *Psychological Assessment of the Elderly.* Edinburgh: Churchill Livingstone.

Pfeiffer, E. (Ed) (1975). *Multidimensional Functional Assessment: The OARS Methodology: A Manual.* Centre for Study of Ageing and Human Development, Duke University, Durham, USA.

Pitt, B. (1987). *Dementia.* Edinburgh: Churchill Livingstone.

Roth, M. and Iverson, L. (Eds). (1986). 'Alzheimer's Disease', in *British Med. Bulletin*, 42(1): 42–50.

Rowland, K.F. (1977). 'Environmental events predicting death for the elderly', in *Psychological Bulletin*, 84(2): 349–72.

Royal College of Physicians (1989). *Care of Elderly People with Mental Illness—Specialist Services and Medical Training.* London: Royal College of Physicians.

Shepherd, M. (1980). 'Mental health as an integral of primary medical care', in *J. of Roy. Coll. of Gen. Pract.*, Nov. 657–62.

Verbrugge, L.M. (1976). 'Females and illness: recent trends in sex differences in the United States', in *J. Health and Soc. Behaviour*, 17: 387–403.

WATTIS, J.P. and HINDMARCH, I. (1988). *Psychological Assessment of the Elderly.* Edinburgh: Churchill Livingstone.

WELLS, L.M. and SINGER, C. (1988). 'Quality of life in institutions for the elderly: maximising well-being', in *The Gerontologist*, 28(2): 266–9.

8   THE QUALITY OF DYING

A well-rounded life should have a beginning, a middle and an end. Not just for the reasons of symmetry but because, though I may be mortal, the social system of which I am part is immortal and my arrival into and departure from that social system are important events which need to be prepared for. Medicine should not confine itself to the prevention of death, any more than family planning should confine itself to the prevention of birth.

Colin Murray Parkes (1978)

Despite the wisdom of these words by Colin Murray Parkes, written in his Foreword to Elisabeth Kübler-Ross's seminal book *On Death and Dying*, much of the practice of modern medicine expresses a basic denial of death rather than a true confrontation of its reality as a part of life. In some respects this is due to the impressive technological advances which makes so many diseases treatable. You will note, however, that I use the word 'treatable' rather than 'curable', and I suggest that the mere application of treatments because they are available, without a realistic appraisal of the quality of the treated patient's life, is a sorry sight. Rather than always attempting to preserve life, there has to be a sensitive and thorough assessment of the likely benefits to be gained from active curative therapy as opposed to proper palliative support, in the form of skilled and compassionate nursing care and effective pain control. One cannot help but recall the words of the nineteenth century British poet, Arthur Clough:

> Thou shalt not kill; but need'st not strive
> Officiously to keep alive.

In fact, many doctors do act with a great deal of care and concern for the quality of their dying patients' lives, but many also admit to viewing death with a personal sense of failure. Olin (1982) found that medical students regarded death as a failure and there is some evidence that people choose medicine as a career because of their own fear of dying. Feifel (1976) reported that medical students fear death more than students not studying medicine and that practising physicians were even more fearful than the medical students. Feifel reasoned that the way to master these death fears is to choose a career in which one can gain power over death by controlling disease and saving lives. This might all sound a little fanciful, but it does provide one of several possible explanations as to why some clinicians '. . . strive officiously to keep alive'. Those doctors unable to confront the fact that certain therapeutic endeavours are doomed, may persist with active therapy. They may find it easier to collude with the desires of both patients and relatives in denying the reality and inevitability of death by the continuance of therapy.

The emotional concerns of the dying person are of interest to us all. Poets, philosophers, scientists, health professionals and lay people have all written about the subject. In this chapter, therefore, I shall adopt a similar approach to that taken in my opening chapter, drawing on literary, philosophical and anecdotal sources as well as those from the scientific medical literature. I shall describe the emotional reactions of dying people and examine the 'quality of dying' in patients suffering from progressive terminal disease.

ATTITUDES TO DYING

The impressive work by Elisabeth Kübler-Ross identified five stages individuals tend to go through before coming to terms with death: 1) denial and isolation; 2) anger; 3) bargaining; 4) depression; and 5) acceptance. There have been a variety of criticisms about her portrayal of attitudes to dying in these discernible stages. One concerns the implicit assumption that it is necessary to pass through all the stages to achieve acceptance of death. Hackett and Weisman (1962), for example, describe the 'middle knowledge' stage, in which patients who realise that they are dying simultaneously refuse to accept death. Engel (1967) suggests that some individuals can cope only by continually denying the reality of impending death. Indeed, such patients, if forced to confront the truth of their situation, become engulfed by an overwhelming and immobilising depression—the so-called 'giving-up-given-up' syndrome.

It seems likely, however, that this represents only a small minority of patients and that the dying are rarely protected from the truth. Studies have shown that most dying people are well aware of the fact that they are terminally sick. For example, Kübler-Ross (1969) interviewed more than 200 dying patients and reported that only three of them maintained denial to the end. Dying people generally feel wretched and can see for themselves the physical deterioration of their own bodies. They also pick up a variety of powerful cues, both verbal and non-verbal, given by friends, relatives and staff. Hollow cheerfulness and optimism about unreachable long-term goals, pitying glances, or stress and anxiety on the faces of loved ones, together with sudden reappearances of friends or relatives not seen for years, all convey a rather obvious message, even if no one has discussed the situation explicitly.

Misguided evasion or frank dishonesty may add considerably to a dying patient's distress and prolong the adjustment process. Patients not given the chance to reveal their fears about impending death are left in anxiety-ridden isolation. If because of the desire by medical staff to avoid distressing disclosures, they fail to make necessary adjustments, such as setting realistic goals and accepting the inevitable, then they are usually unable to enjoy whatever remaining period of life is left. To quote Colin Murray Parkes again (1978):

> Experience has repeatedly shown that if a person is given the opportunity to learn the facts of his case, little by little, at his own pace, and provided he is encouraged to share with others the feelings which these facts evoke, and provided that others are not constantly feeding back to him their own fears, he will move progressively closer to a full realisation of the situation without suffering over-whelming panic and despair.

Concealment of the truth frequently causes anxiety due to uncertainty; it is not uncommon for patients to express relief when this uncertainty is at last dispelled, for many people fear the unknown much more than the truth, however serious that information may be. The fantasies and anxious ruminations of the uncertain dying patient are seldom preferable to a sensitive, empathetic, honest appraisal of what is to be. Patients' fears about dying a lonely, painful death cannot be allayed if no one has raised the topic and provided the opportunity for an explicit discussion. Ivan Lichter (1984), a professor of surgery who has a particular interest in communication with the dying, succinctly conveyed these sentiments:

> Silence may be eloquent . . . (but) . . . If we do not tell, it is not just the diagnosis we have withheld. We have not told the patient that we understand his illness, understand how he feels; we have not told him that we shall support him and that we shall keep him comfortable—this, at a time when he is dependent upon the emotional support of others. It is when the prognosis is bad that there is a need to belong—to family, friends, people.

It is wrong for doctors, nurses and patients' relatives to justify the withholding of an accurate diagnosis and other information on the assumption that the dying always prefer or benefit in some way from pretence. Claims that it is better not to tell the patient because he or she 'couldn't take it' can demonstrate professional arrogance as much as compassion and concern. Relatives who ask the doctor to withhold information on these 'couldn't take it' grounds are usually revealing much about their own fears and reluctance to discuss death, as well as anxiety for their dying relative. It is especially sad to witness when one partner in a relationship refuses to allow the other to be told that he or she is dying. In Lawrence Goldie's words (1982): 'Couples, instead of drawing closer together, wither in each other's arms.'

Facilitating opportunities for partners to discuss death with each other requires tact and skill and doubtless there are exceptional cases when it might not be appropriate, but these exceptions are rare. There is evidence to show that couples need this help. Hinton (1980) interviewed 80 married dying patients and found that 62 of them had discussed the fact that they were dying. It was interesting to note that of these, 85 per cent had spoken about death to the previously unknown interviewer, only 35 per cent had spoken to a member of the medical staff and even less, six per cent, had discussed the subject with a spouse.

We have already seen, in previous chapters, the importance that social support from family and friends plays in maintaining the quality of life of sick people. Medical personnel who collude with relatives of dying patients in an attempt to sustain the myth of immortality, are abrogating their responsibility to assist the patients through the stages that may be necessary to achieve the sort of calm acceptance that will give their patients a more serene and dignified death. Furthermore, the stress and strain of being unable to talk about death leaves much 'unfinished business' which relatives bitterly regret later on. It also denies patients the opportunity of the emotional support from loved ones which they so badly need at this time. In another empirical study of 101 patients with inoperable cancer and their families, Gerle et al. (1960) recorded the emotional difficulties experienced up until death. Half of the group had been told, together with their families, the truth of their prognosis. In the remaining group only the physicians and families knew the full facts and patients were shielded from the information that they were dying. Although the initial emotional distress was greater for the families who were told the prognosis simultaneously with the patients, during the whole period of time from diagnosis to death the emotional upset was greatest for the families in the 'shielded' patients group.

Not everyone, of course, has the sort of personality characteristics which make it likely that he or she would ever view death with calm acceptance. The obituary columns in the newspapers are full of phrases suggesting a fighting spirit: 'battled with illness bravely', 'fought courageously', 'never gave up', etc. This battlefield metaphor can also be seen in Robert Browning's poem, Prospice.

I was ever a fighter, so—one fight more,
    The best and the last!

I would hate that death bandaged my eyes, and forbore,
    And bade me creep past.

The relatives of dying patients often encourage this fighting
spirit. Consider Dylan Thomas' (1966) entreaties to his dying
father:

> Do not go gentle into that good night
> Rage, rage against the dying of the light.

Unfortunately, this sort of encouragement can make some
patients feel extremely guilty if they do not wish to keep
fighting. Worse still, they may see disease progression and
death as a failure on their part for not having battled hard
enough. A young woman dying from breast cancer told me that
the best thing that had happened to her in the previous week
was that she had stopped feeling that she *had* to keep on
fighting. Six months earlier she had visited one of the
alternative cancer therapy centres which encouraged the
notion that one could influence the outcome by adopting a
'fighting spirit' and by adopting a vegetarian diet. She found
the diet unpalatable, especially the vast quantities of carrot
juice that had to be drunk, and she felt too tired to keep
'imaging' the cancer cells being attacked. Fortunately, she had
a close and supportive husband who recognised that the 'fight'
was exhausting rather than helping her. Together they faced
up to the inevitable and found considerable joy and comfort in
this new openness.

> Somehow we seem closer and happier than we've ever
> been now we've stopped pretending what's going to
> happen to me. I've got more time to think about all the
> good things that have happened to us instead of
> concentrating on cancer cells all the time. I've been a very
> lucky person with the job I had, the husband I had and the
> children. It would have been nice to be around for
> grandchildren, but really I've known lots of love in my
> life. Not everyone has that do they? (RH, 1988)

Such sentiments are not uncommon. Consider Bertrand
Russell (1957) who, when contemplating his own death, was
able to comment that:

Happiness is none the less true happiness because it must come to an end, nor do thought and love lose their value because they are not everlasting.

Likewise, Amelia Josephine Burr expressed similar equanimity and calm acceptance in her poem, *A Song of Living*:

> Because I have loved life,
> I shall have no sorrow to die.

But what of those who have not 'loved life'?

Perversely enough, some individuals only appreciate the value of life when they are dying. Even people who have led mundane, unfulfilling lives sometimes experience a new purposefulness and discover reasons for living that had previously evaded them. This reawakening is captured well in the following lines from Walker Percy's *'The Second Coming'* (1980):

> Not once had he been present for his life—
> So his life had passed like a dream.
> Is it possible for people to miss their lives
> in the same way one misses a plane?
> And how is it that death, the nearness
> of death, can restore a missed life?

According to Erikson (1963), we can only face death with equanimity if we can look back at the satisfactory conclusion of various achievements and successes in our lives. If one is unable to do this, then facing death is accompanied by *despair*. One of the most important things anyone caring for the terminally ill can do is to facilitate opportunities for the dying patient to talk and to find this sense of having led a significant and purposeful life. This is not always easy and can tax the ingenuity of the most skilled counsellor, but if Erikson's *integrity* is achieved then patients die in peace with equanimity, rather than in despair.

Depression and Anxiety

I have already spent some time discussing the anxiety aroused by uncertainty, the lack of information, the fear of dying, the fear of pain and fears of abandonment. The quality of death is also affected by depression. The dying person has to contend with a multiplicity of losses: role losses, such as those fulfilled by work, parenthood and within relationships; losses of autonomy, freedom, comfort and privacy; losses concerned with the future, hopes and dreams and aspirations which can never now be realised; losses of bodily function and sometimes body parts. Not surprisingly, the summation of just a few of these can create a black pit of despair. Furthermore, the loss of self-esteem and feelings of helplessness and hopelessness which accompany depression may cause a demise in social skills and therefore impair the willingness of others to provide much-needed social support (Porritt, 1979).

There are some difficult problems with diagnosing depressive illness which could be ameliorated by antidepressant therapy, in patients who are seriously ill. The somatic symptoms of insomnia, appetite loss, extreme lethargy, weight loss, etc, might all be apparent in a dying person who is not depressed. Formal measurement of depression in the dying needs to be refined much more precisely as the symptoms could represent 1) a true psychiatric problem, 2) the illness itself, 3) encephalopathies, for example hypercalcaemia and hepatic failure, 4) possibly even an existential crisis. Kübler-Ross (1978), for example, suggests that depressive symptoms represent a natural turning away from the world when death is imminent. The sort of interventions which might therefore be offered a depressed person with a non-fatal condition may not be appropriate for the dying. Correction of any metabolic imbalances may relieve some of the depression and antidepressant drugs may offer some respite, although they have yet more unwanted side-effects, such as a dry mouth, which dying patients can do without. Skilled counsellors can be effective. In a study by Linn et al. (1982) hospice counselling clearly improved psychological functioning and quality of life in terminally ill patients.

Palliative Care
The verb to palliate is deprived from the Latin—*pallium*, meaning 'cloak'. It used to mean to cloak or hide (which is ironically appropriate if those involved with terminal care engage in cloaking or hiding the truth from patients). Its

modern-day meaning, however, is to lessen the severity of things, such as the pain or suffering in disease.

So far I have addressed mainly the psychological problems encountered by dying patients, but the maintenance of a good quality of life demands that meticulous attention is also paid to adequate symptom control, especially the palliation of pain and discomfort. Table 32, adapted from the impressive and important study by Cartwright and her colleagues, shows the primary symptoms experienced by patients with terminal illness.

TABLE 32

PRIMARY SYMPTOMS FOUND IN TERMINAL ILLNESS

	All other diseases	Cancer
PAIN	66%	87%
INSOMNIA	49%	69%
ANOREXIA	48%	76%
DYSPNOEA	45%	47%
DEPRESSION	36%	45%
CONFUSION	36%	36%
VOMITING AND NAUSEA	30%	54%
DOUBLE INCONTINENCE	24%	36%
BEDSORES	16%	24%
BAD ODOURS	15%	26%
URINARY INCONTINENCE	8%	38%
FAECAL INCONTINENCE	4%	37%
OTHERS	25%	31%

When Cicely Saunders (who was largely responsible for the hospice movement in this country) documented the primary problems of terminal patients with cancer in St Joseph's, she found nausea and vomiting, shortness of breath and dysphagia the top three complaints. Interestingly enough, pain was not high on the problem list, nor was fear of abandonment, showing that these two frequently mentioned complaints can be effectively controlled (1959).

Derek Doyle, the medical director of St Columba's Hospice in Edinburgh, who has a vast experience in palliative care, feels that all the symptoms of terminal illness can be subdivided into three main groups: those which 1) frighten, 2) distress, and 3) isolate patients. The primary symptom which *frightens* patients most is pain.

Pain

Not all dying patients experience pain, although certain diseases are more likely to be painful in their advanced stages, especially metastatic cancer. When chronic intractable pain invades the dying patient's whole world, then her quality of life really is destroyed. Sadly, a review by Bonica (1980) of both American and British data concluded that between 60 and 80 per cent of terminally ill cancer patients experience constant, severe pain. This is especially true of those malignancies with bone and/or nerve involvement. Robert Twycross (1977) has suggested that much of this sort of suffering is unnecessary, as with proper attention to detail and close monitoring it is always possible to relieve the pain of terminal cancer, considerably if not completely.

Another frightening symptom affecting many dying people is dyspnoea (difficulty with breathing). Patients feel convinced that they will suffocate to death and these anxieties tend to exacerbate the dyspnoea. Reassurance that this will not happen is very important, not only for the patient, but also the relatives, who may also feel extremely frightened in the presence of someone with severe dyspnoea.

One of the symptoms which *distresses* patients most is incontinence. Table 32 shows that well over a third of all cancer patients experience the indignity and humiliation of urinary and/or faecal incontinence. In a study by Doyle (1982), the carers of 25 per cent of the male patients dying at home, who had double incontinence, had received no help at all from any home nursing organisation. In such a situation it is hardly surprising that many of these unfortunate people also had to suffer the miseries of bed sores. In these circumstances it is clear that the quality of life for the unfortunate carer is substantially impaired, as well as that of the patient.

One of the symptoms which *isolates* patients most is odour, either from their wounds or fungating tumours, as a result of their incontinence, excessive sweating, or from halitosis. You may recall from Chapter 3 that lung cancer is responsible for more deaths than cancer at any other site; bronchial tumours often produce an exceedingly offensive odour which sometimes cannot be remedied. The aptly named 'cess-pool' halitosis is usually found in people who have delayed gastric emptying or stomach cancer. Patients are profoundly embarrassed by halitosis and are aware that it isolates them further from their loved ones. The trauma of witnessing your own body 'rotting' before your eyes, as happens with fungating tumours, is bad enough; having to live constantly with the smell and to see the disgust on the faces of others is almost too awful for most of us to contemplate. Again, this is a situation where skilled palliative care teams can dramatically improve the quality of patients' lives. Failure to assist patients suffering from these distressing problems adds to their anxiety and to the difficulties of relatives who wish to be loving and supportive. To quote Derek Doyle (1986):

> Odour from fungating tumours, the badly kept colostomy, septic bedsores, incontinence or the poor laundry also holds back visitors, embarrasses those close at hand, prevents the loving couple from sleeping in the same bed and destroys their sexual life. Halitosis occurs in more than 20 per cent of patients and is a cause for them to shun visitors, have no more to do with their spouses and ask to be in single rooms; often it is something we can reverse—the causes are clearly defined and the treatment so simple.

States in life worse than death

Is there a threshold point between a satisfactory quality of life and an unacceptable one, whereby people would decline life-preserving therapy? One feels intuitively that there must be (unless one has a religious faith or philosophical orientation precluding such deliberations), yet specifying precisely just what that threshold point should be is difficult. We could all list items of daily living, physical and psychological functioning which make up our own personal quality of life, and doubtless there would be considerable overlap between the perceptions and priorities of different individuals. Sometimes the relatives of an incompetent patient, such as one who is unconscious, are asked to make decisions about the continuance of life support systems which involve likely quality of life judgements. Recently there has been controversy concerning 'living wills', in which people can make a legal document stating that they wish for no heroic measures to be taken to extend their lives in certain prescribed situations.

Unfortunately, imagining what one's quality of life might be in different states is not the same thing as experiencing that state. The ability to adjust and adapt, exhibited by certain individuals facing appalling situations, is what makes us such successful members of the animal kingdom. Nevertheless, people do have their own basic heuristics for determining when death is a more attractive prospect than continued life. For example, few people would wish to remain in vegetative-like states, in chronic uncontrollable pain or permanently dependent on a ventilator. In an interesting study, Starr *et al.* (1986) found that there was a significant correlation between the perceived quality of life and the desire for cardio-pulmonary resuscitation, when they asked elderly people to consider the option of resuscitation following a stroke which left them disabled, or unable to speak and unable to care for themselves.

On the other hand, Danis and her colleagues (1988) interviewed patients who had survived intensive care and found little correlation between quality of life and willingness to undergo intensive care again if necessary. The assessment of quality of life used in her study was the Norburn Functional Status and Quality of Life Test (Norburn, 1987). This rather general measure could well be too insensitive to pick up the elements of quality of life which become of uppermost importance to patients needing life-preserving or extended care. Furthermore, the subjects studied were those patients who had not only survived intensive care sufficiently to return home, but also they represented those capable of being interviewed. The authors themselves admit that 'the functional status and perceived quality of life of these patients may not have been low enough to provide negative preferences for treatment'.

What is important to consider when looking at the conflicting results of the Starr *et al.* and the Danis *et al.* studies is the fact that what one might feel was an intolerably poor quality of life when viewed from a position of health, might not match up with the value placed on life when one has been or is seriously ill, despite its apparent poor quality to an outsider. I will discuss this issue a little further in Chapter 9, when describing the health economist's view of quality of life.

What do dying people need to enhance the quality of life?

Fortunately, not everyone dies miserably, alone and suffering with intractable pain; many of us will be granted a peaceful, unobtrusive death. Those who are not 'lucky' enough to die in their sleep or following a mercifully short, relatively symptom-free illness can have the quality of death considerably enhanced if given proper palliative care. This chapter has described the problems of dying people under two main headings: physical difficulties and psychosocial difficulties. To some extent, this dichotomy of problems is artificial, as both are inextricably linked with each other. However, I shall for the purposes of clarity summarise briefly the needs of the dying which affect the quality of their death under these two headings.

PHYSICAL NEEDS

1   *Effective symptom control, especially of pain*

The aim of a narcotic drug is to relieve pain adequately and to prevent its return. It is indefensible to limit the dosage of such drugs or the frequency of their administration out of concern that patients will become addicted. Hospice experience has shown that patients who are given satisfactory pain relief, far from becoming addicted, seem to require less medication. Once the fear of pain returning is countered, so is the perception of pain. Although pain is feared most by patients, it is an easier symptom to control than nausea and vomiting, which affects at least 30 per cent of dying patients. Some of this can be corrected with anti-emetic drugs. Presenting small quantities of food a little more imaginatively and at appropriate times can also help.

2   *Proper attention to hygiene*

I have already described the distress caused by foul odours from incontinence, infected or fungating wounds and halitosis. The quality of the dying person's life can be dramatically improved by a good laundry service and such things as aerosols in the sick room. No patient gains comfort from false reassurances that they do not smell offensive when they themselves are able to perceive the odour and can witness the expressions on the faces of others.

3   *Good medical and nursing care*

Many of the frightening, distressing and isolating symptoms of terminal illness can be correlated by good basic care. Hairbrushing, proper washing, regular changes of dressings and clean bedclothes can help patients feel more attractive and more human, and furthermore may ameliorate some of the symptoms. The prospect of food is nauseating to someone with an unchanged dressing on a fungating wound, for example. Pain is substantially increased in a patient with infected bed sores. With imagination and attention to detail, many of the physical problems inflicted on the dying can be made more tolerable.

PSYCHOLOGICAL NEEDS

1   *Honesty*

I have argued that patients and their relatives benefit from an honest discussion about their situation. This permits them to make necessary adjustments and furthermore encourages them to have more faith in the integrity of their medical carers. Reassurance that symptoms will be adequately controlled needs to be matched with action. A patient told that he or she will not suffer pain, who is then not given sufficient analgesia, is unlikely to be reassured by the doctor who later claims that dyspnoea does not mean that he or she will suffocate.

2   *Time*

Patients experience a wide variety of feelings about their inevitable, approaching death. Even if they do not go through the stages outlined earlier, in some clear order, most will experience anger, frustration, fear, despair and acceptance at different times. They need time to express these feelings. Cicely Saunders' entreaty to *listen* to patients, rather than *talk* to them, is important. 'The real question is not "What do you tell your patients?", but rather, "What do you let your patients tell you?"'

3 Comfort and Compassion

It is often possible to provide physical comfort which can also convey emotional care and concern for a dying person. Merely touching someone gently or smiling can bring about both physiological and psychological benefits. Linn and Linn (1986), who have demonstrated the benefits of good counselling, acknowledge that:

> Talk may not be necessary—the comfort of having someone who cares nearby cannot be overestimated. Touching the person lightly on the arm or shoulder can convey one's feelings and reassure the person that he or she is touchable and that communication and understanding exist even at this most basic level.

4 Humour

It is not disrespectful or insensitive to be cheerful when dealing with the dying. Indeed, sombre faces and speaking in hushed tones can make the dying patient feel even more depressed. Cassem and Stewart (1975), in a thoughtful paper, offer some cautions about 'self-styled professional death and dying freaks whose main interest appears to be finding a terminal patient with whom they can discuss death', usually as a means of resolving their own difficulties about the subject. Cassem and Stewart quote a woman in hospital with metastatic breast cancer undergoing chemotherapy. She was apparently argumentative and abusive towards the staff. Later she explained to her doctor: 'I know that I was impossible, but every single nurse who came into my room wanted to talk to me about death. I came there to get help, not to die, and it drove me up the wall.'

5 Facilitation of help and support from the patient's family and friends. The quality of a dying person's life is profoundly

affected by the attitudes of those closest to them. Time spent helping and supporting relatives is an important part of the total care of patients. Some writers have described how impending death demands that patients become existentialists and this is relevant in the context of encouraging friends and relatives to be available in the here and now for patients. Slaby and Glicksman (1985) expand this point:

> Only the moment is guaranteed, and the quality of that point in time determines the quality of their life. If a friend says he/she will drop by some day in the vague future, it has less meaning than the friend who rushes to the bedside to talk, to feel and to touch.

This chapter has adopted a somewhat different approach from that in earlier chapters. I have not really attempted to discuss any formal measures of quality of life applicable to the dying. Although bad practice is obvious, it is difficult to evaluate the impact that tender, loving and competent care has on the quality of dying. As John Hinton (1972) aptly observed:

> We emerge deserving of little credit; we who are capable of ignoring the conditions which make muted people suffer. The dissatisfied dead cannot noise abroad the negligence they have experienced.

Death can be a merciful release from suffering, a tragic event, or the peaceful consequence of a well-spent life.

> And considering the thousand doors that lead to death do thank my God that I can die but once.
> Sir Thomas Browne, *Religio Medici*, 1643

None of us can predict accurately which of the 'thousand doors' we will have to travel through, or the quality of that passage.

References

BONICA, J. (1980). 'Cancer Pain', in Ajemian, I and Mount, B. (Eds), *The RVA Manual on Palliative/Hospice Care*. New York: Arno Press.

CARTWRIGHT, A., HOCKEY, L. and ANDERSON, J.L. (1973). *Life Before Death*. London: Routledge & Kegan Paul.

CASSEM, N.H. and STEWART, R.S. (1975). 'Management and care of the dying patient', in *Int. J. Psychiat. in Med.*, 6: 293–304.

DANIS, M., PATRICK, D.L., SOUTHERLAND, L.I. *et al.* (1988). 'Patients' families' preferences for medical intensive care', in *JAMA*, 260: 797–802.

DOYLE, D. (1982). 'Domiciliary terminal care', in *J. Roy. Coll. Gen. Pract.*, 32: 285–91.

DOYLE, D. (1986). 'Symptom Control: An Overview', in Turnbull, R., *Terminal Care*. London: Hemisphere Publishing Corporation.

ENGEL, G.L. (1967). 'A psychological setting of somatic disease: The "giving-up-given-up" complex', in *Proc. Roy. Soc. Med.*, 60: 553–5.

ERIKSON, E.H. (1963). *Childhood and Society*. New York: W.W. Norton & Company.

FEIFEL, H. (1976). 'Toward Death: a Psychological Perspective', in Schneidmen, E.S. (Ed), *Death: Current Perspectives*. Palo Alto, California: Mayfield Publishing Co.

GERLE, B., LUNDEN, G. and SANDBLOM, P. (1960). 'The patient with inoperable cancer from the psychiatric and social standpoints', in *Cancer*, 12: 1206–17.

GOLDIE, L. (1982). 'The ethics of telling the patient', in *J. Med. Ethics*, 8: 128–33.

HACKETT, T.P. and WEISMAN, A.D. (1962). 'The treatment of the dying', in Masseman, J.H. (Ed), *Current Psychiatric Therapies 2*. New York: Grune & Stratton, pp. 121–6.

HINTON, J. (1972). *Dying*, 2nd ed. Harmondsworth: Penguin Books.

HINTON, J. (1980). 'Whom do dying patients tell?' in *BMJ*, 281: 1328–30.

KÜBLER-ROSS, E. (1978). *On Death and Dying*. London: Tavistock Publications.

LICHTER, I. (1984). 'Communication', in Doyle, D. (Ed), *Palliative Care: The Management of Far Advanced Illness*. Beckenham, Kent: Croom Helm Ltd.

LINN, M.W., LINN, B.S. and HANIS, R. (1982). 'Effects of counselling for late stage cancer patients', in *Cancer*, 49: 1048–55.

LINN, M.W. and LINN, B.S. (1986). 'Caring for the terminal patient', in Stoll, B. (Ed), *Coping with Cancer Stress*. Dordrecht, Netherlands: Martinus Nijhoff Publishers.

NORBURN, J., PATRICK, D.L., BERESFORD, S.A. *et al.* (1987). 'Functional status and perceived quality of life among older persons', in *Proceedings of the 21st Public Health Conference on Records and Statistics*. Washington, DC: National Center for Health Statistics.

OLIN, H.S. (1982). 'A proposed model to teach medical students the care of the dying patient', in *J. of Med. Education*, 47: 564–7.

PARKES, C.M. (1978). 'Psychological aspects', in Saunders, C.M. (Ed), *The Management of Terminal Disease*. London: Edward Arnold.

PERCY, W. (1980). *The Second Coming*. New York: Farrar, Straus & Giroux, London: Secker & Warburg.

PORRITT, D. (1979). 'Social support in crisis: Quantity or quality?' in *Soc. Sci. Med.*, 137: 715–21.

RUSSELL, B. (1957). *Why I am not a Christian*. London: Allen & Unwin.

SAUNDERS, C. (1959). 'The problem of euthanasia', in *Nursing Times*, Oct: 960–1.

SLABY, A.E. & GLICKSMAN, A.S. (1985). *Adapting to Life-threatening Illness*. New York: Praeger.

STARR, T.J., PEARLMAN, R.A. and UHLMANN, R.F. (1986). 'Quality of life and resuscitation decisions in elderly patients', in *J. Gen. Intern. Med.*, 1: 373–9.

TWYCROSS, R.G. (1977). 'Value of cocaine in opiate-containing elixirs', in *BMJ*, 2: 1348.

9 THE HEALTH ECONOMIST'S VIEW OF QUALITY OF LIFE

As we have seen in previous chapters, advancements in medical science have provided us with technologies which permit the treatment of previously fatal diseases and conditions. Perversely, this means that more sick people are now competing for rapidly shrinking financial resources; consequently, even curable disease sometimes goes untreated. The insoluble economic problem of infinite health needs competing for finite financial resources, has led to a variety of utility approaches to measuring health-related quality of life, being incorporated with more basic economic analyses in the hope of providing a fairer means of distributing health care funds. Particularly prominent has been the development of QALYs, or quality adjusted life years. Readers unfamiliar with the language used in 'QALY talk' might find it useful to refer to Table 33.

There has been much confusion amongst some clinicians as to the means by which QALYs are determined. It is irritating to those of us concerned with quality of life assessment in its broadest sense to hear people discussing QALYs as though they are synonymous with the quality of life evaluation discussed in previous chapters of this book. In this chapter I shall look at the theoretical basis and experimental evidence for QALYs and consider the relationship that QALY research has with the measurement of the quality of life of individuals.

Increasingly, clinicians are being asked to justify their health care interventions (especially high cost procedures such as coronary artery bypass grafting) in terms of QALYs (Williams, 1985). Some health authorities have started to use QALY analysis as a means of determining resource allocation (Gudex, 1986). For different disease states, quantitative data such as increased survival and qualitative data concerning disability

TABLE 33
QALY Language

Cost-benefit analysis—health outcome and costs expressed in monetary units

Cost-effectiveness   —health outcome and costs expressed in non-monetary units

Cost-utility   —special case of cost-effectiveness which includes expressed preference for health states

Well-years   —equivalent of a year of completely well life, free of dysfunction, symptoms and health related problems

QALY   —quality adjusted life year. Combination of mortality, morbidity and function (on theoretical line, from dead ⟶ healthy) with quality of life value or UTILITY with increased time of survival resulting from treatment

and distress are all combined with basic economic data, for example the cost of surgical procedures or drug therapy, to provide a calculation of the theoretical cost per quality adjusted life year gained. Thus the central premises underpinning QALY philosophy are the stark economic facts that health demands are infinite and the NHS finances are increasingly limited; a monetary valuation of life utilising various decision theory models is therefore a rational and efficient means of allocating the scarce available resources.

There are, of course, endless political, moral and ethical arguments for and against this viewpoint. Some people maintain that there are resources available to meet needs and that the budget put aside for health care is set at an arbitrarily low level for political reasons. From a moral and ethical perspective there are some interesting dilemmas: a utilitarian approach to the distribution of scarce medical resources *might* result in the majority of the population being better off, but *demands* that others will be considerably worse off. In terms of maximising benefits for the elderly, for example, a utilitarian decision might justify the provision of resources for hip replacements, but at the cost of ignoring altogether anyone requiring renal dialysis, or long-stay institutional care for Alzheimer's Disease. A judgement is being made in such situations which denies individuals the right to *equal* consideration; their lives are considered expendable for the good of others. It is not even clear whether the right to *equal* consideration is fair in moral terms. People who are sicker presumably have greater needs. Thus a morally appropriate criterion for determining the allocation of resources should be based on principles of *equity*, not equality.

This argument presupposes that principles of equality alone will not be sufficient morally to ensure that the distribution of health care resources is either fair, or meets needs. Equity means that like needs should be treated equally, but that unlike needs require an unequal distribution of resources in favour of the most needy.

Such philosophical arguments are important to consider, given the current political climate in which the *laissez-faire* market economy reigns supreme. Consumers of all sorts of goods and services in this country are competing in a system which guarantees social inequality. Health care resources are becoming increasingly susceptible to the market forces which apply to other consumer goods. The Government White Paper on the reorganisation of the NHS, published in 1989, exemplifies this philosophy; if implemented it is likely that the cost-effectiveness of treatment will be the primary imperative determining the provision of health care services, rather than health care needs.

I have chosen to discuss these sensitive and important issues right at the beginning of this chapter in order to encourage the reader to consider the implications that the points raised later have for an *individual's* quality of life.

The utility or decision theory approach to measuring quality of life

Utility theory provides a normative rational model of how decisions are arrived at under conditions of uncertainty. In other words , utility is a general concept for assessing the value that a given individual may place on the consequences of different courses of action. This approach has been applied to health-related quality of life by employing measurement techniques such as standard gamble, time trade-off and various rating scales. These measurement techniques provide a numerical value between zero and one which indicates the desirability of different health states or the quality of an individual's life at a given moment.

Foremost in this field of research is Torrance (1972), and much of his work has been used in the application of cost-effectiveness and cost-utility analysis to health care in North America. He initially worked on the 'gambles' different people would take or risk for improvements in health state and used these data to determine the value of different treatments. Unfortunately, this approach proved too complex for many subjects to understand, so Torrance moved on to develop the time trade-offs (TTO) method (Torrance, 1986). His TTO technique required people to choose between different options in different health state scenarios: that is, remaining in a clearly defined state of ill-health which would lead to death at a specified time, or living in a different state of health which would result in death at another time. Study subjects were asked to make adjustments to these time intervals until they felt indifferent to the choices offered. A schematic model of the application of a TTO approach to a chronic disease state preferable to death can be seen in Table 34. The numerical values between zero and unity that subjects placed on the desirability of different health states derived by this TTO method have been combined with prognostic information about patients who either received or were not given treatment for different disease states. The value of various health care activities could then be measured in terms of the quality adjusted life years gained by the intervention concerned.

Among the many possible criticisms of the Torrance approach are the assumptions that health states are chronic and that death is the worst possible outcome. Also, there is little room in this classification system for the very important psychosocial variables affecting quality of life, as the scenarios for TTO tend to emphasise the physical dimensions. More recent work by Torrance (1982) has described a multi-attribute

TABLE 34

TIME TRADE-OFF FOR A CHRONIC HEALTH STATE PREFERENCE TO DEATH
(after Torrance)

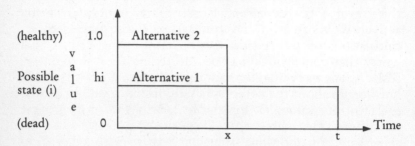

preference value for state i is given by $hi = x/t$

classification system in which six key attributes—physical, emotional, sensory, cognitive, self-care and pain—are used to describe health state. Although more complex analyses are required to determine scale values, the multi-attributable utility theory can be measured using the TTO technique already described.

Loomes and McKenzie (1989) have pointed out another potentially important criticism: the assumption that individuals are 'prepared to sacrifice some constant proportion of their life in order to achieve a given improvement in their health status, irrespective of the absolute number of years that remain'. In other words, is it reasonable to assume that someone who may view ten years of excellent health as equivalent to 20 years in their current state of less than perfect health, would therefore regard two years of excellent health as equivalent to four years in their current state of health, and so forth? There is some experimental evidence to contradict this assumption. For example, McNeil *et al.* (1981), looking at trade-offs between quality of life, in particular speech loss, and survival in treatment for laryngeal cancer, found that their subjects were only prepared to trade survival for improvements in health status if the absolute length of time without perfect speech was greater than five years.

Finally, QALYs determined by TTO methods are not always compatible with QALYs derived using other approaches, such as the psychometric valuations of health states developed by Rosser and her colleagues, which will be described later. Buxton *et al.* (1987) point out that care must be taken as '. . . the use of TTO values and Rosser matrix values are being actively advocated in the context of "cost per QALY" calculations on either side of the Atlantic, there must be a worry that conclusions may be affected by the use of values scaled in one way rather than another.' Torrance (1986) himself has worries about the potentially serious implications that the use of utility values has for specific health states for resource allocation. He states that '. . . these values should be remeasured on additional subjects, perhaps with other techniques, to improve the confidence in the overall result'.

Another approach based on decision theory is that of Kaplan and Bush (1982). They integrate mortality and morbidity data to express states of health in terms of equivalents of well-years of life. If, for example, a woman dies aged 35 following a road traffic accident, when she might well have expected to live until the age of 80, then that accident has 'cost' 45 life years. If, hypothetically, 1,000 35-year-old women, all of whom might have lived until 80, die annually in traffic accidents, then it could be said that 45,000 life years have been lost. Not everyone dies following an accident. Let us suppose that 500 women are left seriously disabled following the accidents and are as a consequence experiencing a very poor quality of life. If the disability is such that quality of life is diminished by 0.75 over the course of a year, than $500 \times 0.75 = 375$ well-years are being lost annually. A rehabilitation programming might improve mobility for 100 of those women, bringing a benefit of 0.25 over a year for each individual, or a 'saving' of 25 well-years for the 100 who all improve. A cognitive behaviour therapy program, on the other hand, may relieve the depression anxiety and overall sense of well-being for 250 of the women, producing a benefit of 0.15 well-years over one year, or $250 \times 0.15 = 37.5$ well-years for the whole group. Cognitive behaviour therapy seems to produce more well-years than the rehabilitation program, so if resources are scarce and provided that it did not cost more in monetary terms, then cognitive behaviour therapy would be the most cost-effective and beneficial therapy to be funded.

These sorts of decision models do theoretically provide a rational framework within which to make efficient use of limited funds, but there are many problems, especially if effectiveness is measured using a single indicator. In Chapter 6 I discussed the fact that analgesia might well reduce joint inflammation and improve mobility of arthritis patients, but this gain has to be offset against the risk and side-effects of long-term drug therapy.

The outcome indicators used as the basis for these supposed gains and losses in well-years must be looked at more carefully. Kaplan and Bush, with their research colleagues, have tried hard to produce a comprehensive measure of health status for their health decision model. They looked at a variety of ways in which different diseases and disabilities affected functioning and organised these findings under three main headings: mobility (e.g. housebound, special care unit, etc.); physical activity (e.g. walking, in wheelchair, etc.); and social activity (e.g. working, needs help with self-care, etc.) (Bush 1983). Almost any disease state can be classified into a well-state from these steps and scales; for example, an arthritic person could be at home, walking with physical limitations and having help with self-care. However, not everyone with problems and symptoms is necessarily dysfunctional. Kaplan et al. (1976) have a large classification system for symptoms and problems to use with the functional scale, which has some positive as well as negative weightings—for example, being on a diet for health reasons scores positively, wearing glasses is negatively weighted.

Using a standardised questionnaire, people can be placed on a defined level of wellness in terms of function and symptoms. Evaluating where this places them in terms of a continuum from death (0) to completely well (1) requires another step, that is a judgement or preference for these different well-states. Kaplan et al. (1976) took random samples of people and gave them 400 case scenarios to rate in terms of preference, from most desirable to least desirable state.

This all starts to sound rather complex, so let me describe a hypothetical example of a man housebound with angina, who could walk around with some physical limitation, but was clearly restricted in terms of the work he could do. Using the standardised questionnaires described earlier, this man might have a 'well-state' value of 0.5549. His primary symptom, i.e. chest pain, would require an adjustment of –0.0382, but the restricted diet and effective drugs he was taking mean another adjustment of +0.1124. Hence this man's quality of well-being score is:

$$0.5549 - 0.0382 + 0.1124 = 0.6291$$

In other words, the people involved in determining these items contributing to wellness would deem him as functioning at a level 60 per cent between death and total wellness. If this man's state of health stayed the same for a year, he would be deemed to have 'lost' 0.3709 of a well-year or 37 per cent of a year.

Not everyone stays in the same state of wellness over the course of a whole year, as they may improve substantially or decline. Some disease states are transitory. Consider the case of someone dying with gastric cancer. On any given day his state of wellness might be exactly the same as someone with a severe bout of food poisoning. The health decision-making policy requires a means of assessing and incorporating the expected well-life expectancy or utility. Using a further equation, the well-life expectancy can be determined. So now we have a score made up of the morbidity, mortality and social desirability of different functional states and a means of measuring the outcome of treatments and interventions in terms of the savings in years of life. One year of life free from disability and health related symptoms and problems constitutes one well-year or QALY.

A rather different approach to the valuation of quality of life can be seen in the work of Rosser and her various collaborators in the United Kingdom (Rosser and Kind, 1978; Kind, Rosser and Williams, 1982). They base their QALY valuations on a matrix of illness states defined on two dimensions of disability and distress. Table 36 shows this matrix and Table 35 the classification of illness states. As QALYs in this country tend to be based on Rosser and Kind's valuations rather than those of Torrance, or the Bush and Kaplan well-years, I shall describe

TABLE 35

CLASSIFICATION OF STATES OF ILLNESS

DISABILITY

(extent to which patient is unable to pursue activities of normal person at time which classification is made)

1 No disability.

2. Slight social disability.

3 Severe social disability and/or impairment of performance at work. Able to do all housework except heavy tasks.

4 Choice of work or performance at work severely limited. Housewives and old people able to do light housework only but able to go out shopping.

5 Unable to undertake any paid employment. Unable to continue any education. Old people confined to home except for escorted outings and short walks and unable to do shopping. Housewives only able to perform a few simple tasks.

6 Confined to chair or to wheelchair or able to move around home only with support from an assistant.

7 Confined to bed.

8 Unconscious.

DISTRESS

(describing patient's pain and/or mental disturbance and/or reaction to disability)

A No distress
B Mild
C Moderate
D Severe

After Rosser, 1976

TABLE 36

Rosser's Valuation Matrix

Disability rating	Distress rating			
	A	B	C	D
I	1.000	0.995	0.990	0.967
II	0.990	0.986	0.973	0.932
III	0.980	0.972	0.956	0.912
IV	0.964	0.956	0.942	0.870
V	0.946	0.935	0.900	0.700
VI	0.875	0.845	0.680	0.000
VII	0.677	0.564	0.000	-1.486
VIII	-1.028	not applicable		

Fixed points: Healthy = 1; Dead = 0

in detail how the Rosser and Kind matrix was derived.

The eight levels of disability and four levels of distress in Rosser's classification system permit 29 possible combinations with which to describe different illness states. There are three theoretically possible combinations which are not included, as it is assumed that unconscious people cannot experience mild, moderate or severe distress. Rosser and Watts (1972) found that, with minimal training, doctors in a general hospital setting could reliably classify more than 2,000 patients using this system. However, there is not always an obvious means of ordering the various combinations of distress and disability in terms of severity. Is VII, A (confined to bed in no distress) a worse state to be in than IV, D (choice of work or performance at work severely limited, etc., experiencing severe distress? I am sure that most readers will find this a difficult judgement to make.

In a painstaking study, Rosser and Kind (1978) collected individual preference and scaling data from interviews with the six different groups of subjects shown in Table 37. They asked subjects to rank-order six 'marker' cards with typed descriptions of health states incorporating a wide range of the possible disability/distress combinations. Among the many things subjects had to do following the ranking procedure was to specify how many times more ill person in state II was than person in state I, and then discuss the implications that such judgements might have in determining the proportion of resources allocated to people in different disease states—for example, treating one person in a severe state or several people in a less severe state. These tiring and stressful interviews took between one and half and four and a half hours and, according to the authors, 'The subjects found the experience of the interviews both painful and relevant. In general, doctors found it particularly difficult and patients found it rather disturbing.' Test and retest reliability was conducted on only ten of the original subjects, as the others had found it so traumatic and fatiguing. Fifty healthy subjects later rank-ordered the marker cards (without the lengthy interviews) on two occasions to test the reliability of the ranking procedure results.

TABLE 37

The Subjects Interviewed to Rank States of Illness
(*Rosser and Kind, 1978*)

Group 1   10 patients from medical wards

Group 2   10 psychiatric in-patients

Group 3   10 experienced state registered general nurses

Group 4   10 experienced state registered psychiatric nurses

Group 5   20 healthy volunteers

Group 6   10 doctors sufficiently experienced to have gained membership or fellowship of at least one Royal College

Many different analyses were carefully carried out and revealed significant differences between the valuations of doctors, medical patients and medical nurses, although psychiatric patients and their nurses, and medical patients and their nurses, showed closer agreements. The doctors seemed to be particularly sensitive to subjective suffering, a finding which might surprise some people. Unlike any other subject group, the doctors rated I,D (no disability, severe distress) as equivalent to VI,A (confined to wheelchair, no distress). In fact, no other group of subjects showed such a marked response to the distress dimension as did the ten doctors.

I do not dispute the importance of this work or the care exhibited by the authors when conducting the research or analysing their results. My very real concern lies with the fact that these data, based on consensus judgements of a mere 70 people (and sometimes there was little consensus), form the primary basis of most QALY valuations in this country. Whilst such consensus data may help in determining the priorities of health care resource allocation, they have precious little to do with the quality of life of an individual. Particularly worrying is the fact that only 20 patients (ten medical, ten psychiatric) took part in the study. There is little clear evidence that such judgements would bear any relationship to the real judgements that would be made by people actually suffering from illnesses such as cancer, heart disease, arthritis or renal failure. Studies such as that by Sackett and Torrance (1978) have shown that valuations made by patients and healthy volunteers are very different. Decisions about the utility of different treatments and trade-offs between increased survival time, set against possible side-effects, for example, are surely very personal matters. Furthermore, the values ascribed to the health states in the matrix are independent of the time actually spent in that state, or of the experience of other states predating current state.

This is an extremely important point to think about, as the values individuals may place on different health states are invariably set in some sort of context: relative judgements about the past and future health state would almost certainly influence the valuation placed on current state. Consider as an example the value that a person might place on state VI,A (confined to a chair or wheelchair in no distress). If one had previously been in perfect health (I,A) with no disability, state VI,A might be an appalling prospect, especially if this was a state likely to continue for an indefinite period. State VI,A, following minor cosmetic surgery on the foot, might not be viewed as such a terrible prospect because the period likely to be spent in that state is very short. On the other hand, someone who had previously been confined to bed for several years (state VII,A), who, as a result of orthopaedic surgery or some new drug therapy, is now experiencing an enhanced degree of mobility, albeit in a wheelchair, might well put a very much higher value on state VI,A than that given in the matrix.

We just do not know enough yet about the changes in quality of life variables which might cause any given patient either to accept or reject a particular treatment. It may well be possible in the future to conduct the sort of research, with appropriate measurement techniques, that is necessary to enable us to draw up a range of values which most sick people would agree upon. However, the current state of the art does not permit the unequivocal acceptance of QALY data as valid material to be used in the allocation of resources for health care. Without an enormous amount of further carefully executed research, QALYs have very little relevance to the urgent health care needs of sick individuals. Even with this work, computation of QALY values will do nothing for you if you happen to be unfortunate enough to suffer from an 'expensive' disease. This seems even more iniquitous when one considers that certain 'life-saving' or preventative services are provided without question, for example the fire service. How much does air and sea rescue service cost in QALY terms? What is the cost per QALY for pot-holers and mountaineers who need rescuing?

There is evidence that the QALY concept is being misapplied, or at least applied too soon on the basis of very limited data. Some cost per QALY analyses are being applied in health authority resource allocations using QALY values computed from United States research data which may not even apply to an English population (Gudex, 1986). Let me give an example from the work of Gudex and her colleagues— the case of a person dying with end-stage renal disease. There are basically four possible treatments which can be offered someone in this situation: 1) continuous ambulatory peritoneal dialysis (CAPD); 2) hospital haemodialysis; 3) home dialysis; and 4) renal transplant. Gudex and her colleagues attempted to establish cost/QALY generated by the different treatments, together with similar analyses of treatments for upper limb joint replacement, drug therapy in cystic fibrosis and the surgical treatment of scoliosis. (This work was done to assist the North Western Regional Health Authority in determining priorities for resource allocation.)

The first step taken was to estimate quality of life using the classification of illness states of Rosser and Kind already described. Gudex *et al.* did this retrospectively by examining the research literature on the subject of quality of life before and after treatment, *irrespective* of how this had been measured by the originators of the various papers. As far as renal failure was concerned, they state: '*No British study with applicable data was found during the literature search and the studies used were all based on the results from American patients.*' Furthermore, 'Because the follow-up periods in the studies were not sufficiently long to estimate life expectancy without treatment, a *range* (my italics) of survival periods was used.'

Not surprisingly, they found variations between the studies 'due to the difficulty in ascribing categories from two different scales (the National Kidney Foundation Classification and Karnofsky Index), into a third, the Rosser Classification'. It was not very easy to transcribe results into Rosser disability grades. Nevertheless, to determine quality of life, the number of patients found to be in each disability/distress category was multiplied by the valuation from the matrix for that category, added together and a mean derived from the sum. This was done for each study, for each of the four end-stage renal disease treatments, and added to information concerning survival.

However, this figure was not the final one used to indicate the resource allocation priorities. The next step was to work out the cost-effectiveness for each QALY gained by different treatments. Table 38 shows an adaptation of these data. It is clear that kidney transplant is a much better bet in terms of cost-effectiveness than CAPD or haemodialysis, but that none of these treatments are as cost-effective as shoulder joint replacement, so this treatment should have priority in health authority funding. Sadly, shoulder joint replacement does not help in kidney failure. All this is rather bad luck, therefore, for those unfortunate enough to have end-stage renal disease which *can* be effectively treated for some time (albeit expensively) with CAPD, haemodialysis or transplantation. Such treatment might seem more preferable to an individual, despite some limitations in quality of life, than death which is a certain outcome without treatment. It is little consolation to someone dying from renal failure to be told that shoulder joint replacement generates more QALYs, if this means that they cannot then receive life-maintaining haemodialysis.

TABLE 38

Cost/QALY data adapted from Gudex (1987)

Treatment	QALYs per patient	Annual cost per patient	Total Cost	Cost/QALY
CAPD (4 years)	3.4	£12,866	£45,676	£13,434
Haemodialysis (8 years)	6.1	£ 8,569	£55,354	£ 9,075
Kidney transplant (lasting 10 years)	7.4	£10,452	£10,452	£ 1,413
Shoulder joint replacement (lasting 10 years)	0.9	£ 533	£ 533	£ 592

CONCLUSIONS

The utility approaches described all have an intellectual appeal. One could argue that the current manner in which resource allocation is determined is entirely arbitrary, unfair and irrational, but producing a slick-looking graph or impressive tables with lots of numbers on them does not necessarily provide a better system unless the method by which those figures were derived is completely sound. I have problems accepting that the methodology is always appropriate, reliable and valid. Quite small variations in the way in which data is collected can produce big differences, thereby affecting the analysis substantially. Mere application of a complex and sophisticated computation does not automatically convey validity if the data base was inaccurately or inappropriately obtained. One thing is certain: the quality of life of sick people can be adversely affected by health economists and others if an objective in QALY research is to provide data supporting arguments for limiting financial resources in health care for treatments that are effective but expensive.

References

BUSH, J.W. (1983). *Quality of well-being scale: function status profile and symptom/problem complex questionnaire.* University of California, San Diego: Health Policy Project.

BUXTON, M., ASHBY, J. and O'HANLON, M. (1987). *Alternative methods of valuing health states: A comparative analysis based on an empirical study using the TTO approach in relation to health states one year after treatment for breast cancer.* Paper presented to 3rd Annual Meeting of Int. Soc. of Technology Assessment in Health Care. Rotterdam, 21-22 May.

GUDEX, C. (1986). 'QALYs and their use by the health service: Discussion paper'. University of York Centre for Health Economics: 14.

KAPLAN, R.M. and BUSH, J.W. (1982). 'Health related quality of life measurement for evaluation research and policy analysis', in *Health Psychology.* 1: 61-80.

KAPLAN, R.M., BUSH, J.W. and BERRY, C.C. (1976). 'Health Status: types of validity for an index of well-being', in *Health Services Research*, 11: 478-557.

KIND, P., ROSSER, R. and WILLIAMS, A. (1982). 'Valuation of quality of life: some psychometric evidence', in Jones-Lee, M.W. (Ed), *The Value of Life and Safety.* North-Holland Publishing Company.

LOOMES, G. and McKENZIE.L. (1989). 'The use of QALYs in health care decision-making', *Soc. Sci. Med.*, 28(4): 299-308.

McNEIL, B.J., WEICHSELBAUM, R. and PAUKER, S.G. (1981). 'Speech and survival: trade-offs between quality and quantity of life in laryngeal cancer', in *N. Eng. J. Med.*, 305: 982-7.

ROSSER R.M. and KIND, P. (1978). 'A scale of valuations of states of illness: is there a social consensus?' in *Int. J. of Epidemiology*, 7(4): 347-58.

ROSSER, R.M. and WATTS, V.C. (1972). 'The measurement of hospital output', in *Int. J. of Epidemiology*, 1: 361.

SACKETT, D.L. and TORRANCE, G.W. (1978). 'The utility of different health states', in *J. Chron. Dis.* 31: 697-704.

TORRANCE, G.W. (1986). 'Measurement of health state utilities for economic appraisal: a review', in *J. of Health Economics*, 5: 1-30.

TORRANCE, G.W., BOYLE, M.H. and HORWOOD, S.P. (1982).

'Application of multi-attribute utility theory to measure social preferences for health states', in *Oper. Res.*, 30: 1043–69.

TORRANCE, G.W., THOMAS, W.H. and SACKETT, D.L. (1972). 'A utility maximisation model for evaluation of health care programs', in *Health Service Res.*, 7: 118–33.

WILLIAMS, A. (1985). 'Economics of coronary artery bypass grafting', in *BMJ*, 291: 326–9.

SUMMARY AND CONCLUSION

This book has revealed a problematic paradox. No one seriously involved in the scientific measurement of quality of life can doubt the need to develop and refine our assessement tools; if we really want clinical medicine to embrace quality of life variables as valid outcome measures then we must produce good quantitative tools. However, part of the motivation behind my insisting that quality of life assessments are made routinely is a desire to give clinical medicine a more holistic face. The scores and numbers produced from our tests are necessary for statistics, which are, of course, important in providing us with information about what is the norm, emphasising similarities between people and between disease states. Good clinical care should therefore be concerned with measures of quality of life, but beyond this should be aware of and responsive to individual differences and needs. I worry that in taking the straight statistical route we may forget or artificially invalidate some other interesting and important paths and byways. The immeasurable aspects of life which give colour, meaning or purpose may be subtly altered or affected by different treatments; they should not be ignored because we cannot yet find a suitable number with which to tag them.

The efforts of psychometricians to develop scientifically valid means of measuring subjective responses must be matched by parallel efforts to revitalise the practice of a more holistic form of medicine. I would argue that effective patient care demands that adequate attention be paid to the impact of treatment on total well-being, instead of just monitoring the physical effects. Advocating quality of life outcomes does not mean that I support weak methodology and soft science; I applaud rigorous scientific endeavour. In view of the formidable research efforts which have substantially improved the validity and reliability of the measurement of quality of life variables, it is surely no longer possible for any medical 'scientist' to dismiss the results as 'soft' science. Unfortunately, continued outright rejection still does seem to exist, calling into doubt the concept of a caring scientific profession dedicated to helping people to maximise both the quantity and the quality of their lives.

However, doctors are not the only arbitrators in deciding who experiences a quality of life which permits human dignity, overall well-being and the fundamental freedoms and rights due to any individual in a civilised society. Politicians have arguably an even greater responsibility; it is they, after all, who determine priorities and goals when targeting resources. The budgetary cutbacks inflicted on health, education, social services and public spending generally over the past decade are eroding the quality of life of many people. Whilst this book has concentrated on *health*-related quality of life, one cannot ignore the importance of other dimensions which add to its value and quality. Sustained economic and industrial growth, education, security and the environment are all as necessary as health and welfare to overall well-being. Political dogma and ideology have created an unhealthy climate in this country, exerting a deleterious effect on the quality of many people's lives. I have constantly referred in this book to the need for doctors to take a broader view of the impact that their treatments have on their patients; likewise, our politicians need to adopt a similar approach. I shall end with this succinct quote from Wortis (1988):

> Good doctors who give drugs to relieve target symptoms always have to reckon with the secondary losses and side-effects, the risks of tardive dyskinesia, addiction, discomfort, distress, etc., and try to strike a reasonable balance in the cost-benefit ratio. The body politic must now give serious attention to the consequences and side-effects of its currently targeted priorities. Nothing less than drastic revision of these priorities can help our chronic patients and the population as a whole.

References
WORTIS, J. (1988). 'Quality of Life', Editorial in *Biol. Psychiatry*, 23: 541–2.

APPENDIX

Addresses for obtaining tests protected by copyright

Nottingham Health Profile   Galen Research and
Consultancy,
2 Finney Drive,
Chorlton Green,
Manchester M21 1DS.

Information can also be
obtained from:
Professor J. McEwen,
Dept. of Community
Medicine,
University of Glasgow
2 Lillybank Gardens,
Glasgow G12 8QQ.

Profile of Mood States
General Health
Questionnaire

NFER/Nelson Publishing
Co. Ltd.,
Darville House,
2 Oxford Road East,
Windsor,
Berks. SL4 1DF.

Psychosocial Adjustment to
Illness Scale

Clinical Psychometric
Research,
PO Box 619,
Riderwood,
MD 21139,
USA.

Sickness Impact Profile

J.B. Lippincott Co.,
East Washington Square,
Philadelphia,
PA 19105,
USA.

GLOSSARY OF MEDICAL TERMS

ADENOCARCINOMA: cancer—the common solid tumour of surfaces, glands and linings.

AIDS: acquired immune deficiency syndrome.

AGRAPHIA: a form of aphasia in which the sufferer is unable to write in a meaningful manner.

ALEXIA: an inability to read, usually as a result of temporal lobe damage.

ALZHEIMER'S DISEASE: (presenile dementia) progressive disorder of brain cells causing severe impairment of higher mental function.

AMNESIA: memory loss.

ANGINA: cardiac pain brought about by effort.

ANTICIPATORY NAUSEA: a classically conditioned response often seen in patients undergoing chemotherapy, whereby stimuli associated with treatment can elicit nausea and/or vomiting.

ANXIOLYTIC: minor tranquillising drug that relieves anxiety.

APHASIA: inability to speak or understand the spoken word.

APRAXIA: inability to carry out intentional movements.

ARC: an AIDS-related complex usually leading to the full AIDS syndrome.

ATHEROSCLEROSIS: hardening of the arteries.

BASAL GANGLIA: structures within the brain composed of grey matter that help control movement and posture.

BETA-BLOCKERS: antagonist drugs that block the beta-adrenergic receptor, often used to treat hypertension.

CARCINOMA: see adenocarcinoma.

CARDIOTOXICITY: poisioning of the heart, usually by drugs; may be temporary or permanent.

CABG: Coronary artery bypass graft.

CHEMOTHERAPY: drug treatment, usually meaning anti-tumour drugs.

CISPLATIN: an anti-tumour drug.

CNS: Central nervous system.

CORONARY ANGIOPLASTY: stretching of a narrowing of an artery in the heart by introducing a balloon into the groin.

CUSHING'S SYNDROME: the effects of excessive adrenocortico-steroids.

CYTOMEGALOVIRUS: a virus infecting immune-deficient patients, mainly affecting brain, eyes and lungs.

CYTOTOXIC: poisonous to cells.

CVA: Cerebrovascular accident or stroke.

DOPAMINE: a catecholamine neurotransmitter, a deficit of which can produce Parkinsonian symptoms, and an excess of which can produce schizophrenia.

DYSARTHRIA: speech impairment due to loss of muscle control of the vocal tract.

DYSPNOEA: difficulty in breathing.

EMETIC: something that causes vomiting.

ENCEPHALOPATHY: generalised disease affecting the brain.

FIBROSIS: replacement of normal body tissue by scar tissue.

HAEMOPHILIA: hereditary bleeding disorder.

HEPATITIS: inflammation of the liver due to many different causes.

HEPATIC FAILURE: complex disorder of the liver that is usually fatal.

HIV: Human immunodeficiency virus.

HODGKIN'S DISEASE: tumour of the lymphatic tissue.

HYPERCALCAEMIA: excessive calcium in the blood, usually caused by very active malignant tumours.

HYPERTENSION: high blood pressure.

IMMUNOSUPPRESSION: lowering of the body's resistance to infection.

ISCHAEMIA: lack of blood supply to part of the body.

KAPOSI'S SARCOMA: multifocal haemorrhagic tumour common in AIDS.

LORAZEPAM: drug used to alleviate anxiety.

LUMPECTOMY: removal of malignant lump, conserving as much of the surrounding tissue as possible.

LYMPHADENOPATHY: enlarged lymph nodes.

LYMPH NODES: small glands in the body, neck, armpits and groin.

MASTECTOMY: amputation of the breast.

METASTASES: deposits of tumour at a site distant from the primary tumour, also known as secondaries.

METHYLDOPA: drug for controlling high blood pressure.

MENINGITIS: inflammation of the membranes around the brain and spinal cord.

MYCOBACTERIA: a group of slow-growing, drug resistant bacteria, e.g. tuberculosis.

MYELITIS: inflammation of the spinal cord.

MYOCARDIAL INFARCTION: (heart-attack) death of part of the heart muscle due to lack of blood.

MYXOEDEMA: effects of lack of thyroid hormone.

NEUROSYPHILIS: effects of infection of the CNS (*qv*) in syphilis.

NEUROPATHY: defects in movements or sensation due to disease of nerves.

NEUROTRANSMITTERS: chemicals which permit transmission of signals between nerve cells.

NEUROTOXICITY: poisoning of the nervous system.

NORADRENALINE: adrenalin-like substance, also a neurotransmitter.

PARAPLEGIA: paralysis of the lower body and legs.

PARESIS: a state of slight or temporary paralysis.

PERNICIOUS ANAEMIA: failure of blood cell manufacture due to malabsorption of vitamin B12.

PERSEVERATION: pathological repetition of thought, speech or action found in brain damage.

PNEUMOCYSTIS CARINII PNEUMONIA: fungus causing infection in immune-suppressed individuals.

PROPRANOLOL: a useful drug in high blood pressure and some heart disease—see beta-blocker.

PSYCHIATRIC MORBIDITY: psychological complications associated with disease and its treatment, e.g. anxiety and depression.

PSYCHOSIS: severe mental disorder of thought, producing hallucinations and delusions, e.g. schizophrenia, manic-depressive disorder, senile dementia.

RADIOTHERAPY: treatment with ionising radiation.

RESERPINE: a major tranquilliser that used to be a popular antipsychotic.

RETROPERITONEAL: the anatomical area behind the peritoneal sac in the abdomen.

SEROPOSITIVE: antibodies in the blood.

SEROTONIN: another neurotransmitter, sometimes known as 5HT. Has an inhibitory action that may control sleep and have a part to play in depression.

STEROIDS: a group of hormones characterised by a sterol ring in the molecule.

TAMOXIFEN: an oestrogen-blocking agent used mainly in breast cancer.

TARDIVE DYSKINESIA: involuntary distortions of facial movements, often caused by prolonged usage of neuroleptic drugs in the treatment of schizophrenia.

INDEX

AIDS (*see also* HIV)
  ARC–AIDS related complex 115
  children with 122
  definitions 114
  PGL—persistent generalised lymphadenopathy 115
  problems for carers 122–4
  psychological problems 117, 120–2
  quality of life in 119–22
AIMS—*see* Arthritis Impact Measurement Scale
abandonment 23, 24, 81
Acquired Immune Deficiency Syndrome—*see* AIDS
adjustment to illness 21–3, 80, 100, 137, 139
  coping strategies 96, 157–60
ADL—*see* Katz Activities of Daily Living Scale
Alzheimer's Disease 171–3
  pressure on carers 172–3
amputation v. limb salvage 100
analysis—*see* tests
angina 127; *see also* coronary artery disease
anxiety 20–1
  in:
    AIDS 120
    cancer 65, 77, 86–7, 90, 93–4, 99
    cardiovascular disease 132–3
    the dying 192–3

relationship with pain 28
Aristotle 28
arthritis
  Arthritis Impact Measurement Scale (AIMS) 47, 150–1
  definitions of:
    juvenile arthritis 143
    osteoarthritis (OA) 144–5
    rheumatoid arthritis (RA) 143–4
  self-assessment test 148
  treatments 146
atherosclerosis 126–7; *see also* coronary artery disease
Auden, W.H. 75
Avoidance behaviour 24
azidothymidine (AZT, retrovir, zovidarine) 116, 120

Beck Depression Inventory 94
beta-blockers 128
Bland, Hubert 29
body-image in:
  arthritis 149
  cancer 84–5, 92
  breast cancer 61, 98–103
  limb sarcoma 100
  testicular cancer 104–6
Browne, Sir Thomas 201
Browning, Robert 178, 190
Burke, Edmund 28
Burr, Amelia Josephine 192
Burton, Robert 169

CABG (coronary artery bypass graft) 130
cancer
  Hodgkin's disease 89–90, 92
  impact of diagnosis 76–80
  impact of treatments 84–92
  leukaemia 13, 31, 84, 89
  breast 45, 51, 75, 78, 85, 96–103, 191
  bowel 38, 40
  head and neck 86
  larynx 208
  lung 81, 95–7
  testis 31, 84, 89, 104–6
  psychosocial problems 77
  relative survival statistics 75, 76, 95, 98, 104
CAPE—see Clifton Assessment Procedures for the Elderly
CARE—see Comprehensive Assessment and Referral Evaluation
Carrington, Dora 177
categorical scales 41
cerebrovascular accident (CVA)
  incidence 126, 133
  Neimi's stroke questionnaire 135
  quality of life 134–7
  quality of life of carers 136
  speech problems 136
chemotherapy
  adjuvant 90
  cytotoxic 13, 51, 88–90, 98–9, 104
  hormonal 91–2, 99
  palliative 90–1
  side effects of 13, 31, 77, 88–9, 90–1, 95–6, 104
    anticipatory nausea and vomiting 88–9
Clifton Assessment Procedures for the Elderly (CAPE) 163–4, 171

CAPE Cognitive Assessment Scale (CAS) 164
CAPE Behaviour rating scales (BRS) 164
clinical trials 31, 61, 78, 95, 108, 129, 130, 138, 149
Clough, Arthur 186
cognitive behaviour therapy 21, 89, 117
cognitive impairment 88, 119, 128, 134, 138
Comprehensive Assessment and Referral Evaluation (CARE) 164–6, 170
compliance 37
concentration camps 22
coronary artery disease 126
  behaviour modification 128
  drugs used in 128–30
  incidence 126
  myocardial infarction 127–8, 131–3
  surgery 130–1
  Type A Behaviour 127–8
counselling 21
  AIDS 119, 123
  cancer 83–4, 87, 91, 94, 106
  cardiovascular disease 139
  terminal illness 192–3, 200
CRC (Cancer Research Campaign) 11, 75
cytotoxic therapy—see chemotherapy
Cytomegalovirus—see opportunistic infections

Davies, Sir John 21
death, fear of 73, 77, 81–4, 120, 127, 187
decision theory—see utility
dementia 116, 119, 167;
    see also Alzheimer's Disease, cognitive impairment
depression 20, 65

in:
AIDS 121
cancer 65, 77, 86, 90, 93–4, 96
elderly 166, 169, 170
heart disease 132
stroke 134
the dying 192–3
diabetes 36–7
doctors 15–16, 31, 43–4, 49, 71,
    83, 187, 214–15, 222
DSM III 93
dying
    attitudes towards 187–92
    denial by patients 188
    denial by doctors 189
    denial by relatives 190
    physical needs of 198–9
    psychological needs of 199–201
    symptoms of terminally ill 194

economics see QALY
    resource allocation 216
elderly
    Age Concern Survey 179
    effects of bereavement in 176–9
    effect of retirement 174–6
    giving-up given-up syndrome
        162
    income of 175–6
    institutions 180–1
    Multiphasic Environmental
        Assessment Procedure
        (MEAP) 181
    numbers of 170, 174
    personal time dependency
        (PTD) 166
    quality of life of carers 169
    Royal College of Physicians'
        Report 170–1
    sexual activity of 168
    use of ADL with 166
Epictetus 21
European Organisation for
    Research and Treatment of
    Cancer (EORTC) 95
    EORTC questionnaire 95–7
equity versus equality 205–6

FLIC—see Manitoba Cancer
    Treatment and Research
    Foundation Functional
    Living Index: Cancer
factor analysis—see measurement
Functional Status Index (FSI)
    150, 152

Galen 25
General Health Questionnaire
    (GHQ) 41, 57, 60, 94, 157
Gibson Spiral Maze 164
glyceryl trinitrate (GNT)—see
    coronary artery disease
Government White Paper on
    NHS (1989) 206
Guttman scales 42

HAD—see Hospital Anxiety and
    Depression Scale
Hamilton Rating Scale (HRS)—
    see Psychiatric semi-struc-
    tured interviews
haemophilia 115, 122
Health Assessment Questionnaire
    (HAQ) 94, 150, 152–4
Herophilus 19
HIV Human Immunodeficiency
    Virus 115–16
    seropositivity effect on quality
        of life 118–19
    worried well 116–18
    see also AIDS
Hodgkin's disease—see cancer
homosexuality—see sexual
    activity
hospices and hospice care 29, 83,
    193–5
Hospital Anxiety and Depression
    Scale (HAD) 67, 69, 94, 99

hypertension (high blood pressure) 126, 133, 137–9
see also cerebrovascular accident
risks of CHD and CVA in 137
side effects of drug therapy for 137–8, 170

information giving 78–9, 87, 91, 95, 188–90
use of audio-tapes in 80
ischaemic heart disease—see coronary artery disease

Jefferson, Thomas 27
Jenkins Activity Survey 128

Kaposi's sarcoma 116; see also AIDS
Karnofsky Performance Index or Scale 38, 44–6
Katz Index of Activities of Daily Living (ADL) 46–8
Kelvin, Lord 17
Kendrick Battery for the Detection of Dementia (KBDDE) 167
Kendrick Cognitive Tests for the Elderly (KCTE) 167

LASA—see VAS
Lerner, Lawrence 26
Levi, Primo 22
Likert-type scoring 57
liver transplants 32
living wills 197
lumpectomy 99–103

Manitoba Cancer Treatment and Research Foundation Functional Living Index:Cancer (FLIC) 55, 56
Mastectomy 65, 90, 98; see also cancer of the breast
McGill/Melzack Pain Questionnaire (MPQ) 52, 54, 150
measurement (see also test) 17
correlation 44, 46, 49
norms and standardisation 39, 63, 166
reliability 33
coefficient 33
split-test 33
test-retest 33
sensitivity 37
specificity 37
standard error 33
validity
construct 36
content 36
criterion 36
face 35
factor analysis 37, 55
Milton, John 28
mood states 67; see also HAD, POMS
multiple sclerosis 23–4, 45, 70
Mycobacterial infection—see opportunistic infection
Myocardial infarction (heart attack) see coronary artery disease

nausea 85, 198; see also chemotherapy side effects
Nietzsche, Friedrich 22
neurological deficits in:
AIDS 119
beta-blocker therapy 128
the elderly 167, 172 see also Alzheimer's Disease
NHF—see Nottingham Health Profile
Norburn Functional Status and Quality of Life Test 197
Nottingham Health Profile (NHP) 55, 57, 58, 59

Older American's Resources and

Services Questionnaire (OARS) 167
opportunistic infection in AIDS 115
Orchiectomy 104

pain 27–9, 36, 52, 54–5, 78, 82, 94, 99, 159, 194–5, 198
PAIS—*see* Psychosocial Adjustment to Illness Scale
paralysis 24
Percy, Walker 192
Pirsig, Robert M. 17
Plato 20
Pneumocystis Carinii—*see* opportunistic infection
politics and quality of life 18, 218, 222
Present State Questionnaire (PSE) —*see* psychiatric semi-structured interviews
Profile of Mood States (POMS) 67, 68, 95, 100, 105
psychiatric semi-structured interviews
    Clinical Interview Schedule 57, 67
    Hamilton Rating Scale 93–4
    Present State Examination (PSE) 93, 98, 99, 105
psychiatric morbidity 65, 132, 157; *see also* anxiety and depression
Psychosocial Adjustment to Illness Scale (PAIS) 40, 61–4, 100

Quack cures in:
    arthritis 155–6
    cancer 107–9
QALY (quality adjusted life year)
    QALY language 205
    cost benefit 205

cost effective 205
cost utility 205
cost per QALY data 146, 218
well-years 209–216
QL Index—*see* Spitzer's Quality of Life Index
quality of life
    definitions of 17–20
    domains in 19–29
        social 23–5
        occupational 25–6
        physical 26–9
    measurement of 33–74
Quality v. quantity 29, 31–2, 108–9, 149, 186
Quality of Well-Being Scale (QWB) 150, 152, 154
questionnaires (see also tests and measures)
    design of 42–4
    choice of 42–4

radiotherapy 85–8
reliability—*see* measurement
retirement 85–8, 174–6
Rosser
    Classification of States of Illness 212–18
    Valuation Matrix 213
Rotterdam Symptom Checklist (RSCL) 61, 62, 99
Ruskin, John 26
Russell, Bertrand 191

Saunders, Cicely 29, 194, 200
sexual activity 24, 25, 40, 45, 77, 86, 98–9, 104, 132, 168, 198
    fertility 106
    homosexuals 114, 118, 121, 123
    impotence 92, 105, 137
Shakespeare, William 21, 27, 84, 162
Sickness Impact Profile (SIPS)

SIPS (*continued*)
    40, 52, 64–6, 100, 129, 131, 152, 154
Sick-Role 25
social scientists 31, 124
social support 21, 25, 45, 82, 86, 137, 162, 170, 173, 179
Sontag, Susan 82
Spielberger State Trait Anxiety 94
Spitzer Quality of Life Index (QL) 48–50
standardisation—*see* measurement
steroids 91, 149
stigma in:
    AIDS 118
    cancer 77, 80–2
stroke—*see* cerebrovascular accident
surgery 15–16
    effect on quality of life 84–5
    arthritis 146
    cancer 77, 98
    heart disease 130
    hip replacement 65, 146, 154
    renal transplant 216–18
Sydney, Sir Philip 28
syphilis 117

tamoxifen 91–2
tests (*see also* measurement and questionnaires)
    analysis of 70

design 33–9, 55
choice of 40–4
testis—*see* cancer
Thomas, Dylan 191
Torrance Time Trade-Off (TTO) 207–9
    schematic model 208

utility 205
    utility or decision theory 206–11

validity—*see* measurement
Visual Analogue Scales (VAS) 41, 134
    LASA (Priestman and Baum) 51–2, 99
    LASA (Selby) 52, 53
    see also FLIC
vomiting 85, 198; *see also* chemotherapy side effects

Wakefield Depression Inventory 94, 98
WHO—*see* World Health Organisation
Wilcox, Ella Wheeler 23
Wolcot, John 23
Woolf, Virginia 27
World Health Organisation (WHO)
    definition of health 19
    incidence of AIDS press release 115
    performance status 46, 47